THE COMPLETE DIABETICS' COOKBOOK

WENDY SILVER

PHOTOGRAPHY BY
RON LOWRY

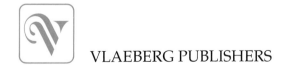

VLAEBERG PUBLISHERS

CONTENTS

FOREWORD □ 3
ACKNOWLEDGEMENTS □ 4
INTRODUCTION □ 5

BREAKFASTS □ 9
SOUPS AND STARTERS □ 13
FISH □ 19
MEAT □ 25
POULTRY □ 33
RICE AND PASTA □ 39
VEGETABLES □ 43
PULSES □ 49
SALADS □ 55
LUNCH AND SUPPER DISHES □ 59
DESSERTS □ 69
BAKING □ 75
SAUCES AND DRESSINGS □ 89
PRESERVES □ 95
SPECIAL OCCASIONS □ 101

METRICATION CHART □ 110
INDEX □ 111

FOREWORD

Despite modern advances, diet remains the cornerstone of both the prevention and treatment of *diabetes mellitus*. In my experience, it is the most difficult aspect of therapy for the health professional to counsel and for the individual with diabetes to understand and comply with. Eating habits are usually an inseperable part of a person's lifestyle and culture. Dietary advice should be part of a sensitive education programme that involves the whole family and aims to deviate as little as possible from customary traditions.

When I was asked to evaluate the text you are about to read, my mind immediately pictured another book proclaiming the benefits of the latest miracle diet. I thought differently after careful study of the text.

The lay-out, advice, scientific approach and gourmet touches to the recipes showed me that Wendy Silver's book is not a simple collection of recipes but an educational experience. Full of varied and interesting ideas, it will add understanding and confidence and make life easier in meeting the individual's particular needs and in improving the eating habits of family and friends.

People with diabetes do not eat "special" foods. Which one of us, wishing to eat well and stay healthy, can afford not to follow advice based on the latest scientific knowledge?

Healthy eating is for everyone!

Professor François Bonnici, MB ChB, MMed, FCP
National President
South African Diabetes Association

ACKNOWLEDGEMENTS

VAL METCALF, who endorsed all the recipes in this book and calculated the exchange values of each, is a Durban-based dietitian, specialising in diabetes and its treatment.
Graduating in 1985 from the University of Natal, Pietermaritzburg, with a B.Sc. in dietetics, Val furthered her studies at the Tygerberg Hospital in the Cape, receiving a diploma in hospital dietetics from the University of Stellenbosch.
During her five years as dietitian at Durban's Addington Hospital, Val was involved in the nutritional councelling of many patients, specifically diabetics. She studied part-time during this period, earning her Honours degree for research into the Comparison of effects of Ensure and Enrich, when used as part of a liquid meal, on postprandial blood sugar levels of non-insulin-dependent diabetic subjects.
Val is a member of ADSA (Association for Dietetics in Southern Africa). For further information about this organisation, contact Jane Badham at P.O. Box 4309, Randburg, 2194.

CAPE SWEETENERS (PTY) LTD. was responsible for all the kilojoule calculations. It is the only company in South Africa which specialises in sweeteners for the food manufacturing industry. It regularly advises food manufacturers on formulations for products suitable for diabetics.

ACCESSORIES for the photographs were kindly supplied by Gabriela's Gifts, Professional Kitchen, Relics and Stuttafords Greatermans, Durban.

INTRODUCTION

WHAT IS DIABETES?
It is estimated that at least three percent of our South African population suffers from diabetes. Genetic factors play a role; but studies have shown overweight to be an important contributing factor. Diabetes **(Diabetes Mellitus)** is a disorder which leads to an excess of sugar in the bloodstream, due to the pancreas failing to produce enough insulin to convert the sugar efficiently into energy. The classic, initial symptoms include great thirst, excessive urination, fatigue, itching and infections of the skin and genitals, blurred vision, menstrual disorders and impotence. There are two major types of diabetes, with marked differences in clinical and physiological characteristics. Treatment for each is different.

Type I or Juvenile Diabetes - Sometimes called ketosis-prone diabetes. It usually becomes evident during childhood or puberty, though it can occur at any age. It accounts for 10 percent of all diabetic cases. The pancreas in this type of diabetic does not produce insulin; daily insulin injections are essential for control. Untreated, the disorder progresses rapidly.

Type II or Maturity-onset Diabetes - The majority of sufferers of this type are obese and, although insulin production in the body is normal or even elevated, it's used less effectively than in the normal individual. This type accounts for the remaining 90% of the diabetic population. Diet is its keystone. About 25% can be treated by diet alone; 25% need a good diet plus insulin; about 50% require a balanced diet, plus tablets. Cure there isn't, control there *is*. The aim of this control is to bring blood glucose levels into the normal range, and to keep them there. This is accomplished through diet, exercise and medication in the form of insulin injections or tablets. Normal blood glucose levels are between 3,5 mmols per litre (65 mg per 100 ml), and 6 mmols per litre (108 mg per 100 ml). In a diabetic, the level of glucose in the blood exceeds this maximum. It must be brought down to within normal limits, and maintained there, to enable the individual to live an active, healthy life.

WHAT IS A DIABETIC DIET?
Eating a proper, balanced diet is important for diabetics *and* non-diabetics. The diabetic diet is fundamentally a healthy one, high in complex carbohydrates and dietary fibre; low in fat. There is no need for the diabetic to be given food different from that eaten by the rest of the family. Indeed, the diabetic may often lead the way for the entire family to change to a healthier way of eating. The diet's energy content should be prescribed to achieve and maintain a desirable body weight. Weight reduction is an important goal in the obese, non-insulin-

dependent diabetic, and has several other spin-offs: improved glycaemic control; increased insulin sensitivity; improved lung function; reduction of elevated blood pressure; reduced risk of surgery, to name but a few. Carbohydrates should provide 55% to 60% of the total daily energy requirement. Wherever possible, fibre-rich, unrefined carbohydrates should be substituted for highly refined, low-fibre carbohydrates. About 30 g to 40 g fibre daily is recommended. The term *dietary fibre* refers to those parts of plant seeds, stems and leaves which cannot be digested by humans. It can be divided into two broad categories: soluble and insoluble. Sources of soluble fibre include oats, fruit, barley and legumes; oat bran and dried beans being particularly good. When mixed with water, soluble fibre forms a gel. This moves along the gastrointestinal tract like a sponge, delaying the emptying of the stomach. This sponge-like behaviour slows the absorption of carbohydrates, and lowers blood cholesterol – both invaluable to the diabetic. Insoluble fibre is found in fruit and vegetable skins, wheat and most grains. It absorbs many times its weight in water, providing bulk and quick passage of wastes through the intestinal tract. Its toning effect on intestinal muscles provides protection against colon cancer. Although there is still controversy over the amount and type of fibre necessary in the diabetic's diet, following the current recommendations *can* improve metabolic control.

Guidelines for adding fibre to the diet include:
☐ increasing fibre intake slowly. Discomfort and flatulence may occur initially, but will dissipate;
☐ eating a variety of foods rich in both soluble and insoluble fibre, wholegrain cereals, fruit and vegetables with skins, wholewheat bread, bran, oats, nuts, seeds, lentils, dried beans and other legumes.

Of the daily energy intake, 12% to 20% should come from protein sources, or about 0,8 g/kg body weight. Too high a protein consumption may place undue strain on the diabetic's kidneys and exacerbate the rate of renal function deterioration. A slightly higher protein/body weight ratio is only acceptable during pregnancy, lactation, or periods of rapid growth in young children and adolescents. Total fat intake should be restricted to less than 30% of the daily energy allowance. Saturated fat should provide less than 10%; polyunsaturated fat less than 10%; mono-unsaturated fat the remainder. Reduced fat intake has a twofold benefit: it reduces the total energy content of the diet; and results in increased insulin sensitivity and enhanced glucose metabolism. Alcohol in moderation poses no great health risk to the diabetic, as long as sensible guidelines are followed. Alcohol provides 29kJ per gram, and contains little in the way of nutrients, so the overweight diabetic should abstain altogether. In the well-controlled diabetic, daily intake should be limited to two glasses of dry wine, one mixed drink, or two beers. Drinks containing large amounts of sugar such as liqueurs and sweet wines, should be avoided. Mixers, such as tonic water, should have a low carbohydrate content. Diabetics should never drink on an empty stomach, and must remember to include the kilojoules in their daily energy total.

ALTERNATIVE SWEETENERS

Simple sugars – brown and white sugar, glucose, dextrose and honey are quickly absorbed into the bloodstream, causing blood glucose levels to rise sharply. That is why these, plus foods high in added sugar – jam, sweets, puddings, cakes, biscuits, fizzy drinks and several canned products should be avoided by the diabetic. The exception is the treatment of hypoglycaemia or insulin reaction,when the blood glucose drops below acceptable levels. It is then essential to eat or drink something sweet to avoid convulsions or a coma. Alternative sweeteners were developed to satisfy the need for sweetness in all of us, young and old, dieter and diabetic, without adding appreciable energy to the diet. Sweeteners fall into two categories: nutritive and non-nutritive. Nutritive sweeteners, such as fructose and sorbitol, provide some energy; while non-nutritive sweeteners are synthetic products which contain no energy, such as saccharin and cyclamate.

Fructose (fruit sugar) has the advantage of tasting sweeter than sucrose (sugar), and is metabolised without insulin, therefore producing less hyperglycaemia. However, it has the same kilojoule content as sucrose, and no more than 50 g a day should be included in the diet. It is also very expensive. Sorbitol has the same kilojoule content as sucrose, but is not as sweet. It is absorbed slowly and passively into the bloodstream, but can cause diarrhoea, abdominal gas and discomfort. The use of special sorbitol and fructose-containing foods for diabetics is not recommended. Many have an increased fat content to make the food more palatable, thereby substantially increasing the kilojoule content. Ideally, non-nutritive sweeteners should have a taste similar to that of sucrose, and no change in taste should take place during cooking or baking. Although perfectly safe to use within normal limits, a long-term, excessive intake of sweeteners may have harmful side-effects, so moderation is of paramount importance. A mix of various types of sweeteners, each with its particular advantages, is recommended in order to distribute any potential risks of over-indulgence.

Saccharin - the best-known non-nutritive sweetener is about 500 times sweeter than sucrose. Because of its bitter after-taste, it's usually combined with cyclamate.

Cyclamate - the least sweet of all sweeteners is usually combined with others for a better taste.

Aspartame - 200 times sweeter than sucrose, it is not suitable for cooking or baking, since prolonged heating reduces the sweetness. Persons suffering from phenylketonuria, an extremely rare disease, must avoid products sweetened with aspartame.

Acesulfame k - one of the latest non-nutritive

sweeteners on the market is 200 times sweeter than sucrose. It has a pleasant taste and long shelf-life, and is often blended with other sweeteners.

Note: Before you decide on which sweetener to use, check the label to find out if it is suitable for baking and cooking. Also read the ingredients' list carefully before you buy. In all this book's recipes, I have used the liquid sweetener, NATREEN, made of saccharin, cyclamate and fructose. Its use has been sanctioned by the SA Diabetes Association and by Val Metcalf, the dietitian who checked the recipes. Whenever I mention "granular sweetener", this is Natreen in powdered form, its ingredients being aspartame and maltodextrine (a type of sugar). This product is not suitable for baking or cooking, and should be used only occasionally by the diabetic, in very small amounts. As Natreen granules have some kilojoule content (0,5 g contain 8,5kJ), this energy value must be taken into account in your daily calculations.

COMPOSITION AND USES OF MARGARINE

According to South African legislation, all yellow margarines must be made from vegetable oils only, with Vitamins A and D added to equal the vitamin content of butter.

Margarine must have a minimum fat content of 80%, the same as butter, the balance made up of 16% water and 4% additives emulsifier, milk solids, preservative (sodium benzoate), flavouring and colouring (Beta-Carotene). A versatile product, it comes in brick or tub form, and can be used for spreading, melting, baking and frying. As soon as the fat content drops below 80%, the product cannot be labelled margarine; it's then called a "spread". A medium-fat spread has a fat content of 50% to 65%, with 35% to 45% water. It can be used for spreading, melting and baking – cakes biscuits and pastries are inclined to turn out hard. It is not suitable for frying, as the water content is too high.

A low-fat spread contains only 35% to 45% fat, and 55% to 65% water. It should be used only for spreading and melting, *not* for cooking, baking or frying. Choose a margarine or medium-fat spread wherever "margarine" is called for in this book's recipes. Only use low-fat spread when specifically called for. Remember, all fats and oils yield the same energy – one gram equals 38kJ. The chief advantage of using margarine as opposed to butter lies in the reduction of saturated fat consumption, *not* in the kilojoule content. Low-fat spreads *do* have a lower gram for gram fat content, but have limited usage.

IMPROVING YOUR RECIPE

When choosing a recipe for a diabetic, there are several important points to bear in mind, and questions you need to ask yourself:

☐ Does the fat content seem too high? If the recipe requires more than 25 ml oil or 30 g margarine/butter for four servings, try halving the amount, and see if it noticeably affects the end-result. Two excellent ways of reducing the amount of fat required for frying or sautéing are:

a) use non-stick spray in a non-stick pan and cook over low heat;

b) cook onion, garlic, etc, in a small bowl in the microwave oven on 100% (High) power, about one minute, or until soft. No fat is needed.

☐ If the amount of fat is justified, drain the food on absorbent kitchen paper towels, and wipe out the pan, before proceeding with the recipe.

☐ Cook fatty meat (such as mince and sausages) the night before and, when cool, refrigerate overnight. The fat will rise to the surface and solidify, making it easy to scrape off with a spoon before reheating.

☐ Steam or bake instead of frying, wherever possible.

☐ Substitute wholegrain products for refined ones, wherever possible. Using wholewheat flour for baked goods tends to give a heavy, close-textured result. Combine white flour with wholewheat for a lighter, more satisfactory product.

☐ Use more vegetables and less meat. Sliced, crumbed brinjal, or large mushrooms cooked in soy sauce, make good meat substitutes.

☐ Can olive-oil be substituted for sunflower oil or margarine without affecting the flavour too much? Or, perhaps use half olive-oil and half sunflower oil? Being a mono-unsaturated fat, olive-oil is the cook's best choice, but sometimes the flavour is too strong for the dish, and it's necessary to use an alternative.

☐ If the fat content of a baked product is halved, will the recipe still work successfully? Trial and error is the only way to achieve the maximum texture and flavour with the least amount of fat.

☐ Can the cheese in the recipe be reduced or omitted? Which cheese can be used with the lowest fat content without spoiling the recipe? If the cheese is the chief source of protein, allow 30 g per person; if not, you can use far less, without compromising on nutritional value.

☐ Instead of cream for thickening or enriching, try potatoes or fresh breadcrumbs in soups and stews; low-fat yoghurt in desserts, purées and mousses; or reduce the liquid by boiling rapidly for a few minutes.

☐ Instead of gravy, make a smooth vegetable purée, chunky mushroom sauce or tangy tomato and onion mixture – probably more tasty, and certainly more healthy than flour-thickened pan drippings!

☐ Will the recipe work with sweetener instead of sugar? Choose recipes which don't have a high flour to sugar ratio, and remember that the method may have to be altered as well. Here again, trial and error is the only way to a successful solution.

☐ Can the number of eggs in the recipe be reduced? Can one use the whites only and omit the yolks? Egg-yolks are high in cholesterol, so limit their consumption to two or three a week. Going through this checklist each time, and with a little experimentation, you will be able to add several more recipes to your repertoire without compromising on health or palatability.

GENERAL HEALTH AND AVOIDING COMPLICATIONS

Diet therapy forms the basis of the treatment of *diabetes mellitus* patients, and good diabetic control within satisfactory body-weight limits will go a long way to reducing the chances of complications. Genes contribute about 70% towards the probability of your developing diabetes. You cannot choose your parents; but there are several factors over which you *do* have control and of which you should be constantly aware:

☐ have your blood-pressure, triglyceride and cholesterol levels checked regularly;

☐ have your eyes tested at least every six months;

☐ don't smoke;

☐ keep alcohol consumption to a minimum;

☐ have your feet checked regularly;

☐ have blood and urine tests done once a year;

☐ have an E.C.G. once a year.

Your doctor and other members of the health-care team – nurses, dietitians and chiropodists are there to advise you, and provide the information, support and technology to enable you to look after yourself and live a normal, healthy, long life.

FURTHER INFORMATION

To keep abreast of the latest research and technology in the treatment of diabetes, and to share your problems and ideas with fellow diabetics, become a member of The South African Diabetes Association. Write to them at P.O. Box 3943, Cape Town, 8000, and they will put you in touch with a branch of the Association nearest to you. Membership will entitle you to free diet information and regular newsletters on the latest happenings, seminars, products, and so on .

EXCHANGE LISTS

Exchange lists at the end of each recipe are lists of foods with similar nutrient composition which are interchangeable within a given diet plan.

Dietitians use these exchange lists to work out daily diets for their diabetic patients, hence their inclusion under each recipe.

The exchange values used throughout this book are based on those of the American Diabetes Association (1988 edition).

For the average diabetic, or health-conscious cook, exchange values are not important, as the nutritional analyses under the recipes will give sufficient pertinent information to calculate his/her daily food intake.

Note: To calculate kilojoules from Calories (Kcal), multiply by 4,2.

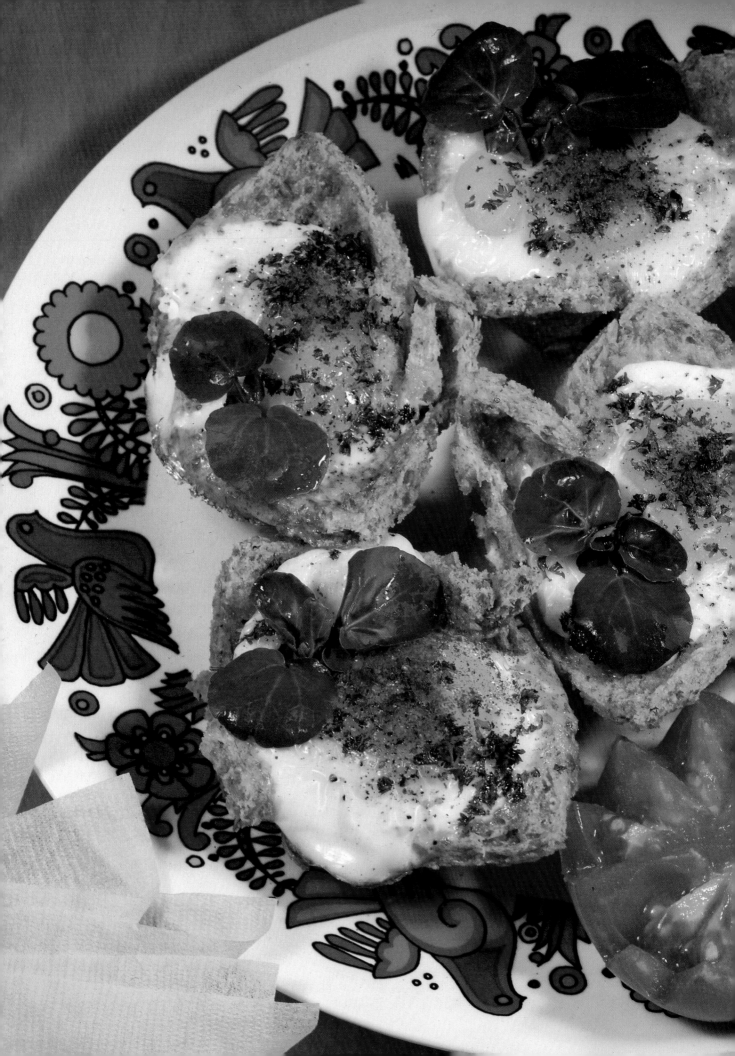

BREAKFASTS

This first meal of the day should be loaded with unrefined, complex carbohydrates (whole grains), which are slowly digested, ensuring a gradual, sustainable level of blood sugar throughout the morning. Fruit, with its fructose and glucose, will act as an instant pick-me-up after the long night hours, and will provide essential vitamins and minerals as well. Although high in cholesterol, eggs are, nevertheless, an excellent source of protein, and should not be excluded from the diet entirely. Keep intake to two or three a week. Breakfast should constitute about one-third of the day's kilojoule intake.

BAKED EGGS

6 thin slices pre-sliced wholewheat bread, crusts
  removed
25 g margarine, melted
25 g (60 ml) low-fat hard cheese, grated
6 medium eggs
20 ml finely chopped parsley
salt and freshly ground black pepper to taste
paprika to sprinkle

Roll bread slices with a rolling-pin until very thin. Use to line muffin pans sprayed with non-stick spray. Brush protruding points of bread with melted margarine. Divide grated cheese between the six pans, break an egg into each. Sprinkle parsley and seasoning over each, bake at 190 °C, about 15 minutes, or until just set. Sprinkle with paprika, serve at once with grilled tomato and watercress.

Serves six

Per serving: 762kJ; 13,9 g carbohydrate; 10,1 g protein; 9,7 g fat;
212 mg cholesterol; 2 g fibre
Exchanges: 1 starch; 1 meat; 1 fat

FISH AND POTATO *FRITTATA*

350 g baby potatoes, scrubbed
10 ml olive-oil
1 onion, thinly sliced into rings
4 garlic chives, finely sliced
180 g smoked trout, skinned, boned and flaked
2 eggs
3 egg-whites
37,5 ml skim milk
salt and freshly ground black pepper to taste

Cook potatoes in boiling, lightly salted water, about 15 minutes or until just tender. Drain, rinse under cold, running water, skin and slice, set aside. Heat 5 ml olive-oil in a frying-pan, sauté onion and chives, two to three minutes, stirring. Add remaining 5 ml olive-oil and potatoes, fry over medium heat until lightly browned. Scatter flaked fish over potatoes. Remove from heat, set aside.
Whisk together eggs, egg-whites, milk and seasoning, carefully pour egg mixture over potato mixture in pan. Cover and cook over gentle heat until edges are set but centre is still slightly liquid, about eight minutes. Place under preheated griller until top is lightly browned and set, one to two minutes. Don't overcook or egg mixture will be tough. Cut into six wedges, serve at once.

Serves six

Per serving: 657kJ; 12,8 g carbohydrate; 13,3 g protein; 5,2 g fat;
93 mg cholesterol; 1,3 g fibre
Exchanges: 1/2 starch; 1 1/2 meat

◄ Baked eggs

MUESLI

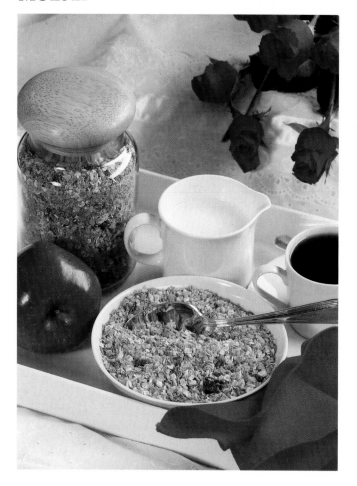

WHOLEWHEAT FRENCH TOAST

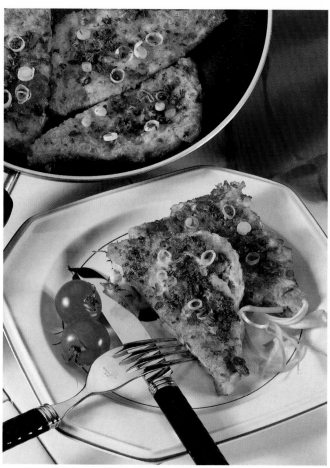

180 g (500 ml) rolled oats
40 g (250 ml) digestive bran
180 g (500 ml) wheatgerm
130 g (500 ml) wheat flakes
120 g (250 ml) sunflower seeds
30 ml nibbed almonds
75 g (125 ml) prunes, stoned and chopped
50 g (125 ml) dried apricots, chopped
50 g (125 ml) non-fat dried milk powder
75 g (125 ml) raisins

Spread out first five ingredients on large baking trays. Bake at 160 °C, about 40 minutes. Add almonds, prunes and apricots, bake a further five minutes. Remove from oven, allow to cool completely. Empty into a large bowl, add milk powder and raisins, stir well. Store in airtight containers. To serve, spoon about 125 ml muesli into a breakfast bowl, add warm or cold water with artificial sweetener to taste, stir well.

Makes about 910 g, or 20 servings of 125 ml each

4 x 12 mm-thick slices wholewheat bread
60 ml skim milk
4 egg-whites
25 ml finely chopped parsley
4 spring onions, finely chopped

Cut bread into triangles, remove crusts. Whisk together milk, egg-whites, parsley and spring onions in a shallow bowl. Dip bread triangles into milk mixture, fry in heated non-stick frying-pan, three to four minutes on each side. Serve at once.

Serves four

Per serving: 681kJ; 19,3 g carbohydrate; 6,8 g protein; 5,8 g fat; 0 mg cholesterol; 8,7 g fibre
Exchanges: 1 starch; 1 fat

Per serving: 374kJ; 14,5 g carbohydrate; 6,5 g protein; 0,6 g fat; 0 mg cholesterol; 2,1 g fibre
Exchanges: 1 starch

GRAPEFRUIT, APPLE AND PEAR MIX

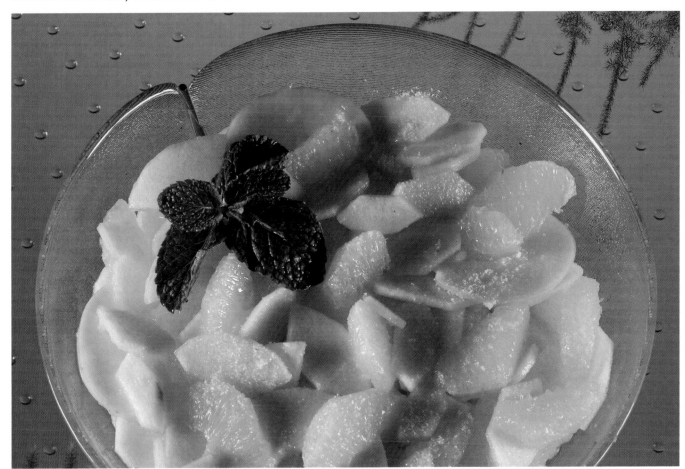

3 grapefruit, thickly peeled, segmented and juice reserved
2 Golden Delicious apples, cored and very thinly sliced
2 pears, peeled, cored and very thinly sliced
granular artificial sweetener to sprinkle

To decorate
mint

Place grapefruit segments with juice in a bowl. Add apple and pear slices, mix gently. Sprinkle with sweetener, cover and refrigerate one hour. Toss again gently, spoon into individual serving bowls. Serve chilled or at room temperature. Decorate with mint.

Serves 10

Per serving: 464kJ; 24,7 g carbohydrate; 0,9 g protein; 0,6 g fat; 0 mg cholesterol; 3,8 g fibre
Exchanges: 1 1/2 fruit

MEALIE-MEAL CRUMPETS

120 g (250 ml) yellow mealie-meal
250 ml boiling water
5 ml baking-powder
8 drops liquid artificial sweetener
1 ml salt
125 ml skim milk
1 egg, lightly beaten

Place mealie-meal in a mixing-bowl, add boiling water, stir well. Leave to stand five minutes. Whisk together remaining ingredients, add to mealie-meal mixture, whisk until a smooth, thin batter is formed. Spray a large, non-stick frying-pan or griddle-iron with non-stick spray, heat well. Drop about 25 ml batter at a time on to the hot surface, spread into a circle about 100 mm in diameter. Cook until bubbles appear on surface and underside is lightly browned, one to two minutes. Turn and cook other side, a further one minute. Transfer to a heated serving platter, cover and keep warm. Repeat with remaining batter, making 12 crumpets in all. Serve warm with Home-made Tomato Sauce (see Page 92), or a little melted margarine.

Serves six

Per serving: 392kJ; 17,4 g carbohydrate; 3,5 g protein; 1,3 g fat; 34 mg cholesterol; 0,7 g fibre
Exchanges: 1 starch

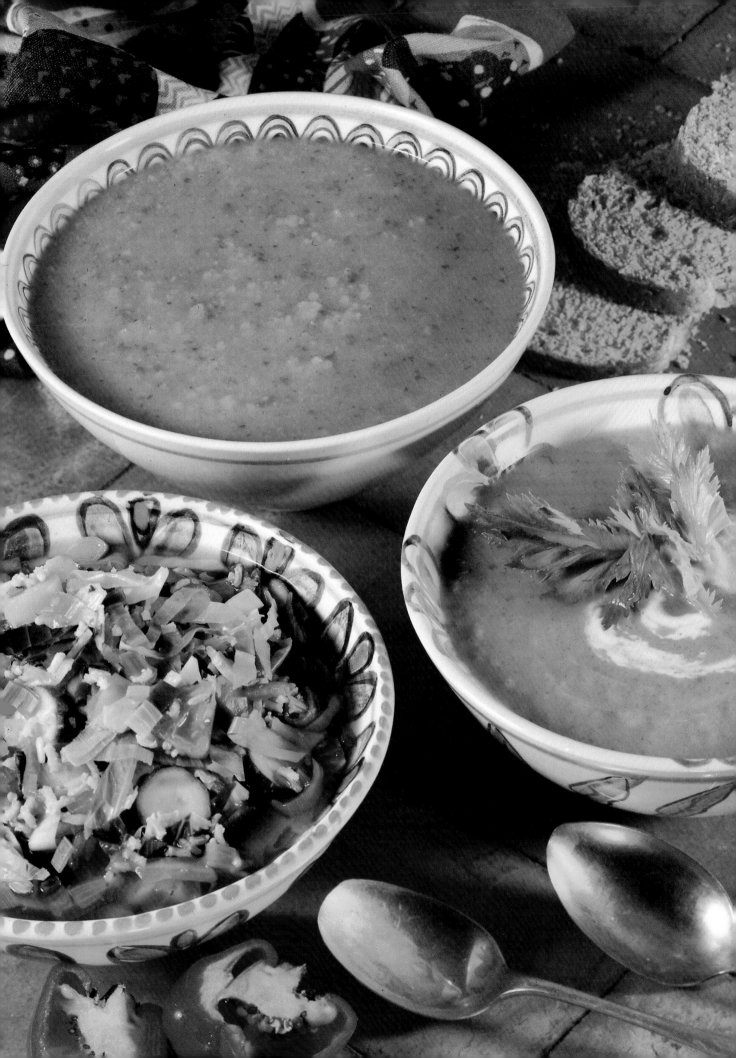

SOUPS AND STARTERS

Soups can be simple starters or sustainable main meals. They can be thick and hearty or thin and light and, if prepared in large quantities, will freeze well for several months. Instructions for making various stocks – the bases for good soups – are included throughout this book. Starters should be served in small portions, just enough to whet the appetite for the meal to follow. If served in larger amounts, they make delicious, quick lunch or supper dishes, accompanied by wholewheat bread, a salad or a few vegetables.

CARROT AND TOMATO SOUP

37,5 ml sunflower oil
2 large onions, finely chopped
1 kg carrots, scraped and sliced
4 large ripe tomatoes, skinned and chopped
1,25 litres home-made chicken stock (see Page 34)
finely grated rind and juice of one orange
salt and freshly ground black pepper to taste
50 ml finely chopped parsley

Heat oil in a large saucepan, add onions and carrots, fry gently five to eight minutes. Remove with slotted spoon, drain on absorbent kitchen paper towels. Wipe out saucepan, return carrot mixture to pan, together with remaining ingredients. Bring to the boil, stirring continuously. Reduce heat, cover and simmer 15 minutes, or until carrots are tender.
Remove from heat, purée in batches in food processor or electric blender. Return to rinsed-out saucepan, heat through, thinning down with a little water, if necessary. Serve hot.

Serves six

Per serving: 754kJ; 21,1 g carbohydrate; 3,6 g protein; 6,8 g fat; 0 mg cholesterol; 8,2 g fibre
Exchanges: 1 vegetable; 1 fat

THICK CELERY SOUP

1 large onion, finely chopped
1 head of celery, trimmed and chopped, including leaves
1 red pepper, seeded and diced
1 green pepper, seeded and diced
30 g chives *or* spring onions, trimmed and chopped
600 ml home-made chicken stock (see Page 34)
125 ml skim milk
salt and pepper to taste

Place all ingredients, except milk and seasoning, in a large saucepan, bring to the boil, stirring continuously. Reduce heat, cover and simmer 30 minutes.
Purée in batches in food processor or electric blender. Return to rinsed-out saucepan, heat through. Add milk and seasoning, simmer 10 minutes. Serve with wholewheat bread.

Serves four

Per serving: 184kJ; 7,2 g carbohydrate; 2,4 g protein; 0,4 g fat; 1 mg cholesterol; 2 g fibre
Exchanges: 1 vegetable

COUNTRY VEGETABLE SOUP

1 onion, finely chopped
2 large leeks, trimmed and sliced
1 small cabbage, finely shredded
4 small baby marrows, trimmed and sliced
2 large ripe tomatoes, skinned and chopped
60 g (75 ml) raw brown rice
5 ml dried sweet basil
3 ml dried tarragon
3 cloves of garlic, crushed
freshly ground black pepper to taste
3 ml celery salt
1,25 litres home-made beef stock (see Page 26)
37,5 ml tomato purée

Place all ingredients in a large saucepan, bring to the boil, stirring frequently. Reduce heat, cover and simmer 30 minutes. Adjust seasoning to taste, serve hot.

Serves six

Per serving: 349kJ; 14,2 g carbohydrate; 2,8 g protein; 0,6 g fat; 0 mg cholesterol; 4,2 g fibre
Exchanges: 1/2 starch; 2 vegetable

◀ Clockwise from top: Carrot and tomato soup; Thick celery soup; Country vegetable soup

SPINACH-STUFFED MUSHROOMS

CHICKEN, POTATO AND SPINACH SOUP

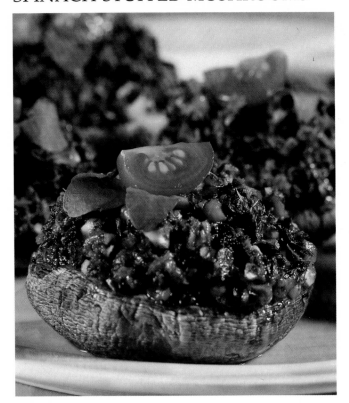

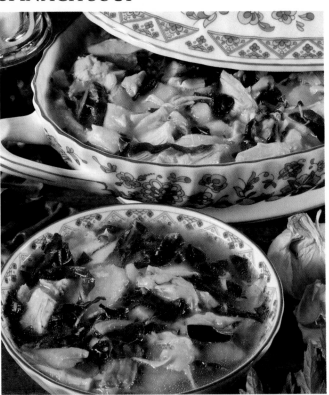

A delightful start to a meal, they may also be served as a vegetarian main meal. Serve two per person, accompanied by seasonal vegetables or a mixed salad, and wholewheat bread.

6 large brown mushrooms, wiped
5 ml olive-oil
1 small onion, finely chopped
1 clove of garlic, crushed
125 g frozen chopped spinach, thawed and thoroughly drained
30 g feta cheese, diced
freshly ground black pepper to taste

To garnish
cherry tomatoes, quartered
watercress

Remove stems of mushrooms, chop stems finely, set caps aside. Heat olive-oil in a large frying-pan, sauté onion and garlic, one to two minutes. Stir in mushroom stems and spinach. Cook one to two minutes over high heat, stirring. Remove from heat, add feta cheese and black pepper. Pile on to mushroom caps, arrange on baking tray. Place under preheated griller, six to eight minutes, until just tender. Serve at once, garnished with cherry tomatoes and watercress.

Serves six

Per serving: 194kJ; 3,4 g carbohydrate; 2,7 g protein; 2,4 g fat; 4 mg cholesterol; 1,4 g fibre
Exchanges: 1/2 vegetable

1,5 kg chicken, all skin and visible fat removed
1 onion, peeled and halved
1 celery stalk, roughly chopped, including leaves
1 bunch of parsley
2 bay-leaves
5 ml cumin seeds
2 ml dried thyme
2-3 cloves of garlic, peeled
8 ml salt
500 g potatoes, peeled and thickly sliced
125 g fresh spinach, finely shredded
freshly ground black pepper

Place first nine ingredients in a large, heavy-bottomed saucepan. Add enough water to cover, about 2,5 litres, bring to the boil. Reduce heat, cover and simmer one hour, or until chicken is tender. Skim off any foam which rises to the surface. Strain liquid through a colander, reserve contents of colander except bay-leaves. Discard all but 1,5 litres of liquid. Pour liquid back into rinsed-out saucepan, bring to the boil. Add potato slices, simmer 10 minutes, remove with a slotted spoon. Purée half potato slices with 250 ml liquid in electric blender or food processor, return to saucepan. Remove meat from chicken, cut into bite-sized pieces, add to saucepan together with remaining potato slices and shredded spinach. Bring to the boil, season with pepper and serve at once.

Serves six

Per serving: 2 373kJ; 17,6 g carbohydrate; 67,4 g protein; 22,7 g fat; 220 mg cholesterol; 2,2 g fibre
Exchanges: 1 starch; 3 meat

CRÊPES AU POISSON *(Fish-filled wholewheat pancakes)*

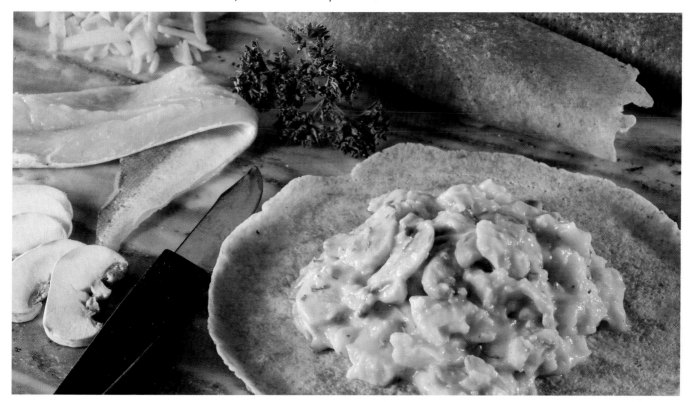

Pancakes make a marvellous emergency meal, besides doubling up as a super starter or pud for a dinner party. Keep a stack of ready-made ones in the freezer, to thaw and use at a moment's notice. Vary the filling to suit the occasion: mushrooms, chicken, sweetcorn or cheese in a white sauce base; savoury mince; tomato, herb and onion mixture – all suitable as a starter or light meal served with salad. For dessert, fill with dried, canned or fresh fruit, and serve with custard.

Wholewheat pancakes
**125 g (250 ml) wholewheat flour, sifted and
  husks replaced**

1 egg	**10 ml sunflower oil**
2 egg-whites	**250 ml skim milk**

Fish filling
300 g frozen white fish fillets, skinned
325 ml water *or* home-made chicken stock (see Page 34)
125 ml dry white wine *or* water
40 g margarine
100 g button mushrooms, wiped and sliced
12,5 ml fresh lemon juice
30 g (60 ml) wholewheat flour
10 ml chopped fresh dill *or* parsley
salt and freshly ground black pepper to taste

To complete
50 g (125 ml) low-fat hard cheese, grated
paprika

Wholewheat pancakes
Place flour in a mixing-bowl, make a well in centre. Beat together remaining ingredients, pour into well, whisk

well until a smooth, thin batter is formed. Cover and leave to stand about one hour.
Coat inside of a small frying-pan with non-stick spray, heat well. Spoon about 50 ml batter into pan, tilting and shaking pan to spread batter evenly over base. Cook until bubbles appear on surface and underside is lightly browned. Turn over, cook the other side. Remove to a warmed plate. Repeat with remaining batter.

Fish filling
Poach fish in water and wine until tender, about 10 minutes. Remove fish from liquid, skin and flake, set aside. Strain cooking liquid, set aside.
Melt 20 g margarine in a frying-pan, add mushrooms, sauté until soft, three to four minutes. Add lemon juice, bring to the boil. Cook over high heat until all the liquid has evaporated. Remove mushrooms from pan, and set aside.
Melt remaining margarine in same pan, stir in flour, cook one minute. Remove from heat, stir in reserved cooking liquid. Return to heat, bring to the boil, stirring continuously. Stir in the dill, mushrooms and fish. Season to taste.
Divide filling between pancakes, roll up. Arrange, seamside-down, in a lightly greased ovenproof dish, sprinkle with cheese and paprika. Bake, uncovered, at 180 °C, 15 minutes. Serve hot, with lemon wedges and sprouts or watercress.

Serves six

Per serving: 1 119kJ; 19 g carbohydrate; 18,1 g protein; 10,9 g fat; 63 mg cholesterol; 3,4 g fibre
Exchanges: 1 starch; 1 1/2 meat; 2 fat

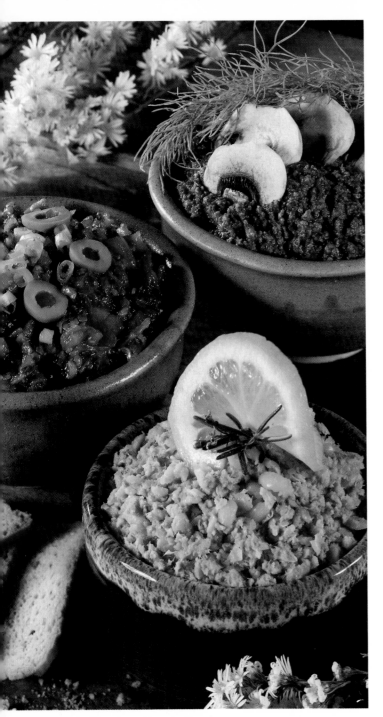

MUSHROOM AND LENTIL PÂTÉ

1 onion, finely chopped
5 ml sunflower oil
200 g large brown mushrooms, wiped and grilled
100 g (125 ml) brown lentils, cooked and drained
60 g smooth low-fat cottage cheese
25 ml chopped parsley
squeeze of lemon juice
garlic salt and freshly ground black pepper to taste
37,5 ml home-made beef stock (see Page 26)

Fry onion in oil until soft. Purée all ingredients in a food processor or an electric blender. Spoon into individual serving dishes, cover and chill well before serving. Serve with lettuce, tomato and Melba toast.

Serves six

KIPPER PÂTÉ

300 g kipper fillets, cooked, skinned, boned and flaked
50 ml smooth low-fat cottage cheese
200 g dried white haricot beans, soaked overnight, cooked and drained
12,5 ml fresh lemon juice
10 ml bottled anchovy sauce
sprinkling of cayenne pepper
salt and freshly ground black pepper to taste

Place all ingredients in an electric blender or a food processor, purée until smooth. Adjust seasoning. Spoon into individual serving dishes, cover and chill well before serving. Serve with lettuce and Melba toast.

Serves six

BRINJAL PÂTÉ

2 large brinjals, wiped
25 ml olive-oil
salt and freshly ground black pepper to taste
juice of one lemon
few drops of liquid artificial sweetener
1 clove of garlic, crushed
25 ml finely chopped parsley

To garnish
onion rings
sliced stuffed olives

Bake whole brinjals in a 180 °C oven, one-and-a-quarter hours. Peel and mash with a fork. Place in a bowl, add remaining ingredients, mix well. Spoon into suitable serving dishes, cover and chill well before serving. Garnish with onion rings and sliced stuffed olives.

Serves six

Clockwise from top: Brinjal pâté; Kipper pâté; Mushroom and lentil pâté

Mushroom and Lentil Pâté
Per serving: 387kJ; 9,8 g carbohydrate; 7 g protein; 1,8 g fat; 2 mg cholesterol; 3,4 g fibre
Exchanges: 1/2 starch

Aubergine Pâté
Per serving: 235kJ; 2,3 g carbohydrate; 0,5 g protein; 4,4 g fat; 0 mg cholesterol; 2 g fibre
Exchanges: 1/2 vegetable; 1 fat

Kipper Pâté
Per serving: 794kJ; 12,6 g carbohydrate; 17,5 g protein; 5,3 g fat; 30 mg cholesterol; 8,6 g fibre
Exchanges: 1 starch; 1 meat

MUSHROOM SOUP

BROCCOLI AND CHEESE SOUP

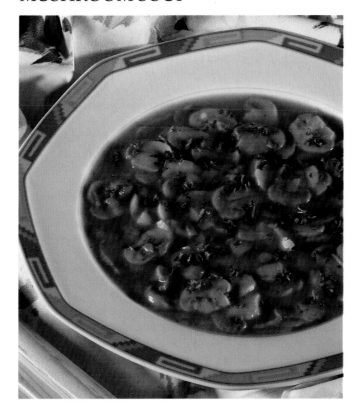

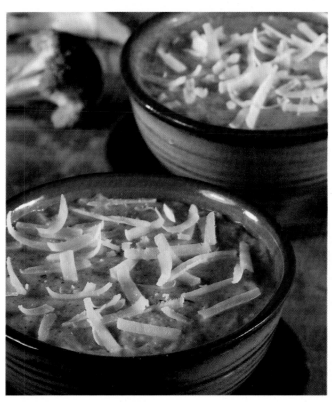

10 g margarine
10 ml sunflower oil
1 large onion, thinly sliced
600 g button mushrooms, wiped and sliced
1,2 litres home-made chicken stock (see Page 34)
125 ml skim milk
25 ml dry sherry (optional)
good grinding of black pepper
25 ml finely chopped parsley

Heat margarine and oil in a large, heavy-bottomed
saucepan. Sauté onion, four minutes, until soft. Add
mushrooms, reduce heat, cover and cook two minutes,
stirring occasionally. Uncover, increase heat. Cook until
moisture has evaporated, and onion is golden brown,
about 10 minutes. Stir continuously to prevent burning.
Remove mushroom mixture, drain on absorbent kitchen
paper towels. Wipe out pan, return mushroom mixture,
add stock, milk, sherry if used, and pepper. Bring to the
boil. Reduce heat, simmer, uncovered, 15 minutes.
Adjust seasoning to taste, and sprinkle with pàrsley
before serving.

Serves six

Per serving: 321kJ; 6 g carbohydrate; 3 g protein; 4 g fat; 0 mg
cholesterol; 1,6 g fibre
Exchanges: 1/2 vegetable; 1/2 fat

2 large heads of broccoli, broken into florets
5 ml olive-oil
2 onions, finely chopped
2 cloves of garlic, crushed
250 ml low-fat plain yoghurt
40 g (80 ml) wholewheat flour
750 ml home-made vegetable or chicken stock
   (see Pages 44 and 34)
3 ml salt
1 ml freshly ground black pepper
1 ml cayenne pepper
3 ml dried origanum
2 ml dried thyme
100 g (250 ml) low-fat hard cheese, grated

Bring a large saucepan of salted water to the boil, cook
broccoli eight to 10 minutes, drain and set aside. Heat
oil in a small frying-pan, sauté onions and garlic, three
minutes. Remove with a slotted spoon, drain on
absorbent kitchen paper towels.
Purée broccoli and onion mixture in an electric blender
or food processor until smooth, set aside.
Combine yoghurt and flour in a saucepan, beat with a
wire whisk. Add stock, seasonings and herbs, whisking
continuously. Reduce heat, cover and simmer for
20 minutes. Add broccoli purée and 75 g (190 ml)
cheese, stir until cheese has melted. Remove from heat,
ladle into warmed soup bowls, top with remaining
grated cheese, serve at once.

Serves six to eight

Per serving: 568kJ; 11,3 g carbohydrate; 11,1 g protein; 4,8 g fat;
10 mg cholesterol; 3,3 g fibre
Exchanges: 1 vegetable; 1/2 starch; 1/2 meat

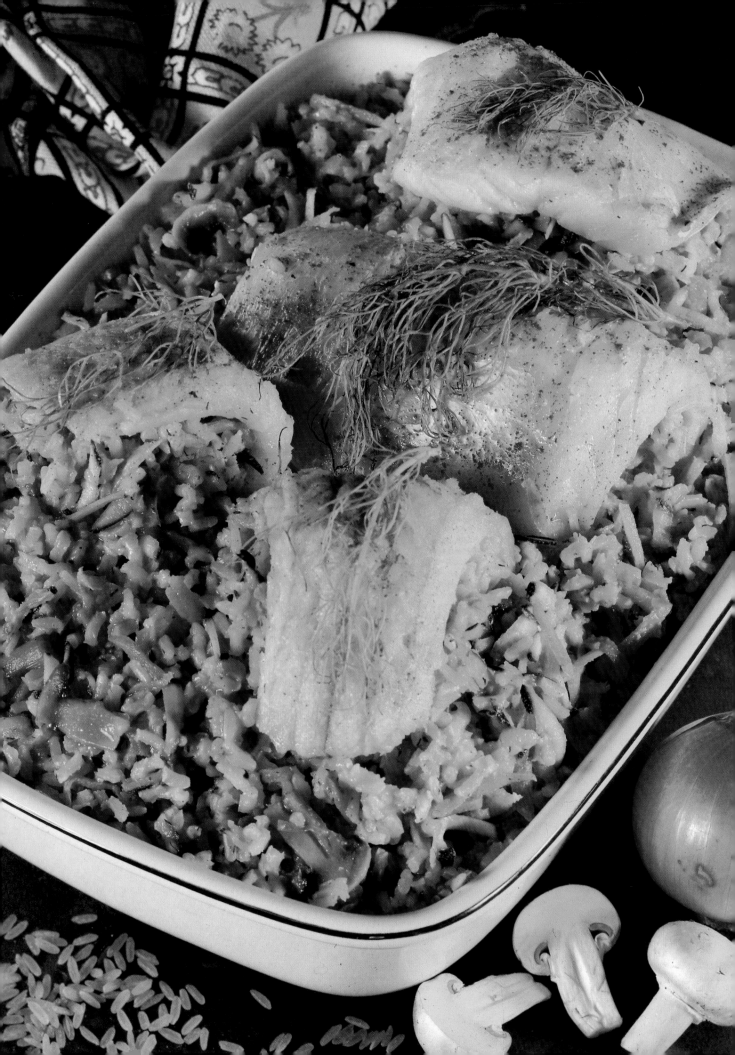

FISH

Provider of one of the most concentrated sources of high-quality protein, fish is also rich in many vitamins and mineral salts. Low in calories and cholesterol, it forms a valuable addition to the diabetic's diet. Leaner varieties are prized for their modest amounts of kilojoules, while the fattier types contain fish oil which lowers the level of blood fats, and discourages the blocking of arteries. Octopus, squid, prawns and crab – high in cholesterol – have been omitted.

RICE-STUFFED KINGKLIP

1 large onion, chopped
100 g button mushrooms, wiped and sliced
12,5 ml sunflower oil
750 ml home-made fish *or* chicken stock (see Pages 20 and 34)
125 ml skim milk
10 g (20 ml) cornflour
5 ml dried dill
400 g (500 ml) raw brown rice
3 carrots, scraped and grated (about 500 ml)
4 baby marrows, trimmed and grated (about 500 ml)
1,2 kg kingklip fillet, cut into four pieces
salt and freshly ground black pepper to taste
paprika
fresh dill *or* fennel to garnish

Sauté onion and mushrooms in heated oil, in a large, heavy-bottomed saucepan, three to four minutes. Add stock, stir well. Combine milk and cornflour, add to saucepan with dill, bring to the boil, stirring. Add rice, return to the boil. Reduce heat, cover and simmer about 25 minutes or until all liquid has been absorbed and rice is tender. Remove from heat, add carrots and baby marrows, stir well. Cover and leave to stand five minutes. Season kingklip with salt and pepper. Spread about half of the rice mixture over base of a lightly greased 200 mm by 300 mm ovenproof dish. Fill kingklip fillets with remaining rice mixture, fold in half and arrange on rice mixture in dish. Sprinkle with paprika, cover with foil, shiny side inside, and bake at 180 °C, 25 to 30 minutes, or until fish is tender. Garnish with dill and serve at once, with freshly squeezed lemon juice.

Serves eight

Per serving: 1 345kJ; 24,9 g carbohydrate; 33,7 g protein; 7,6 g fat; 59 mg cholesterol; 3 g fibre
Exchanges: 1 vegetable; 1 1/2 starch; 3 1/2 meat

SOLE WITH CRUMB TOPPING

half an onion, finely chopped
half a green pepper, seeded and diced
12 g (50 ml) fresh brown breadcrumbs
25 ml finely chopped parsley
25 ml finely chopped fresh coriander
3 garlic chives, finely sliced
3 ml salt
2 ml lemon pepper
25 g margarine, melted
6 small dressed soles

Herbed tomato sauce
125 ml tomato juice
2 ml dried origanum
2 ml dried basil
1 ml ground coriander
3 ml freshly squeezed lemon juice
few drops liquid artificial sweetener
lemon slices to garnish (optional)

Combine first eight ingredients in a small bowl, stir in melted margarine. Arrange soles in a single layer in a lightly greased shallow ovenproof dish, or roasting-pan. Top with crumb mixture. Bake, uncovered, at 180 °C, about 20 minutes, or until fish flakes easily when tested with two forks.

Herbed tomato sauce
Combine tomato juice, herbs, coriander and lemon juice in a small saucepan, bring to the boil. Boil until slightly reduced. Add sweetener to taste. Serve soles with herbed tomato sauce, brown rice and a salad.

Serves six

Per serving: 536kJ; 3,7 g carbohydrate; 17,5 g protein; 4,4 g fat; 48 mg cholesterol; 0,5 g fibre
Exchanges: 2 meat; 1 fat

◄ Rice-stuffed kingklip

HOME-MADE FISH STOCK

Can be made very economically, using left-over fish, bones and trimmings; but be sure not to use oily fish as the flavour will be too strong.

1 kg white fish, e.g. Red Roman, Stumpnose, Grunter
2 large onions, finely sliced
2 celery stalks, sliced
2 small carrots, scraped and sliced
500 ml dry white wine *or* water
25 ml fresh lemon juice
1 large leek, split, washed and sliced
2 cloves of garlic, crushed (optional)
5 stems of parsley
3 sprigs of thyme
2 bay-leaves
5 black peppercorns
2,25 litres water   Exchanges: free

Step 1:

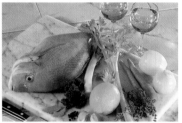

Collect all ingredients.

Step 2:

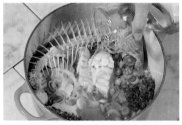

Place all ingredients in a large, heavy-bottomed saucepan, adding water last. Bring to the boil, skim off any scum which rises to the surface. Reduce heat, simmer gently 20 to 30 minutes.

Step 3:

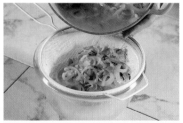

Strain stock through a fine sieve. Discard contents of sieve. Allow stock to cool completely. Cover and store in refrigerator for up to three days, or pour into suitable containers and freeze for up to two months.

Makes about two litres.

20

POACHED HAKE WITH MUSHROOM SAUCE

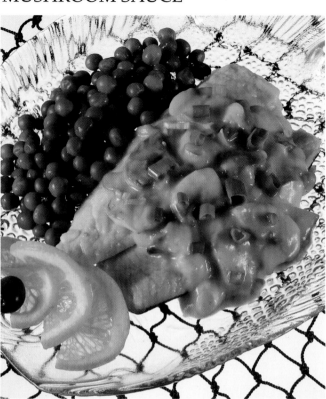

1 onion, peeled and quartered
1 carrot, scraped and diced
1 bay-leaf
3 ml dried thyme
600 ml water
400 g frozen hake fillets, skinned
25 g margarine
12 g (25 ml) wholewheat flour
100 g button mushrooms, wiped and sliced
3 ml finely grated lemon rind
salt and freshly ground black pepper
25 ml chopped chives
lemon slices and black olives to garnish

Bring onion, carrot, bay-leaf, thyme and water to the boil in a large frying-pan. Boil, uncovered, 10 minutes. Add fish, cover and simmer gently 10 to 12 minutes, until fish is tender and flakes easily when tested with a fork. Remove fish, set aside, keep warm. Strain liquid, set aside. Make a white sauce with margarine, flour and reserved liquid, cook until thick. Stir in mushrooms, lemon rind, seasoning and 12,5 ml chopped chives. Cook, stirring, one to two minutes. Spoon over fish, sprinkle with remaining chopped chives. Serve at once, garnished with lemon slices and black olives, and with mashed potato and green peas as accompaniments.

Serves four

Per serving: 795kJ; 6,2 g carbohydrate; 20,4 g protein; 8,4 g fat; 38 mg cholesterol; 1,9 g fibre
Exchanges: 1/2 vegetable; 2 meat; 1 fat

BAKED HADDOCK WITH TOMATOES AND BABY MARROWS

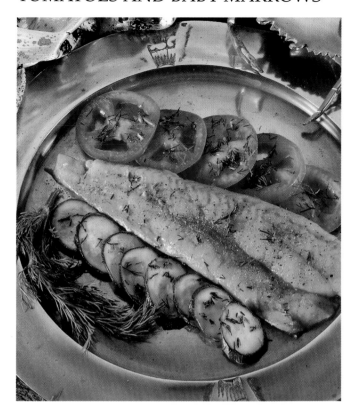

TUNA-STUFFED POTATOES

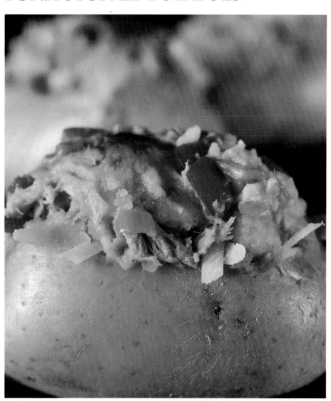

600 g frozen haddock fillets, skinned and thawed
freshly ground black pepper
12,5 ml chopped fresh dill
2 cloves of garlic, crushed
500 g ripe tomatoes, sliced and seeded
3 baby marrows, trimmed and diagonally sliced
salt to taste
10 ml olive-oil

Arrange haddock fillets, overlapping slightly, in base of a lightly greased, rectangular ovenproof dish. Sprinkle with pepper and half the dill and garlic. Cover with layer of tomato slices, then with layer of baby marrows. Sprinkle remaining dill and garlic over baby marrows, add salt to taste. Drizzle olive-oil over surface. Cover with foil, shiny side inside, and bake at 200 °C, 20 to 30 minutes, or until fish flakes easily when tested with two forks. Serve at once.

Serves six

4 large even-sized potatoes, scrubbed
25 ml finely chopped spring onions
25 ml finely chopped red pepper
185 g can tuna in brine, drained and flaked
25 g (60 ml) low-fat hard cheese, grated
25 ml low-fat plain yoghurt
salt and freshly ground black pepper to taste

Bake potatoes at 200 °C, one hour, or in microwave on 100% (High) power, four minutes for each potato, until tender. Cut a 6 mm-thick slice off top of each potato, scoop out pulp, leaving shell intact. Set shells and pulp aside. Coat inside of a non-stick frying-pan with non-stick spray, place over medium heat. Add spring onions and red pepper, sauté one minute. Add tuna, sauté a further minute. Remove from heat, turn into a small mixing-bowl. Add potato pulp, 30 ml cheese, yoghurt and seasoning, stir well.
Stuff potato shells with mixture, top with remaining cheese. Place under preheated griller until heated through and cheese melted. Serve at once, with a green salad.

Serves four

Per serving: 511kJ; 3,3 g carbohydrate; 18,7 g protein; 2,9 g fat; 54 mg cholesterol; 1,6 g fibre
Exchanges: 1 1/2 vegetable; 2 1/2 meat

Per serving: 729kJ; 23,9 g carbohydrate; 14,4 g protein; 1,4 g fat; 14 mg cholesterol; 2 g fibre
Exchanges: 1 starch; 1 1/2 meat

TUNA FISH CAKES

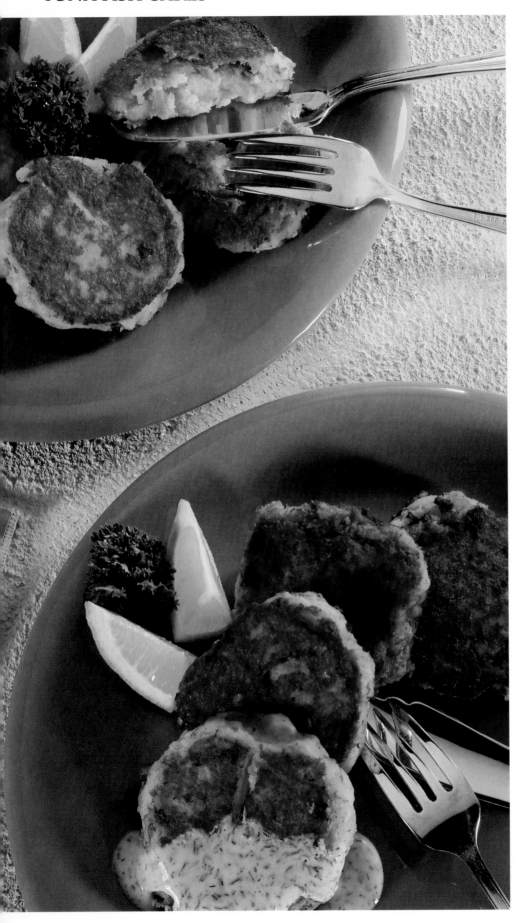

Equally tasty eaten cold, these fish cakes may be stored in the refrigerator for two to three days in a sealed container, or frozen for up to two months.

3 large potatoes, boiled, skinned and mashed
1 large egg
1 egg-white
3 spring onions, finely sliced
185 g can tuna in brine, drained and flaked
60 ml finely chopped parsley
12,5 ml fresh lemon juice
12,5 ml low-fat plain yoghurt
few drops of Tabasco sauce
3 ml salt
freshly ground black pepper to taste
10 g margarine
10 ml olive-oil

Dill sauce
125 ml low-fat plain yoghurt
30 ml chopped fresh dill *or* 10 ml dried dill to taste

Chill mashed potatoes at least 30 minutes, or overnight. Whisk egg and egg-white, beat in potatoes, spring onions, tuna, parsley , lemon juice, yoghurt, Tabasco sauce, salt and pepper. Chill mixture at least 30 minutes, or overnight if required. Heat margarine with olive-oil in a large frying-pan. Using hands, form mixture into 12 patties about 50 mm in diameter and 12 mm thick. Mixture is soft, so handle carefully. Fry, four at a time, until golden brown underneath, about four minutes. Turn and cook other side, a further three to four minutes. Drain on absorbent kitchen paper towels, keep warm. Serve with Dill sauce.

Dill sauce
Combine yoghurt and dill, cover and chill at least 30 minutes, or overnight, before serving.

Serves six

Per serving: 618kJ; 13,7 g carbohydrate; 10,5 g protein; 5,1 g fat; 47 mg cholesterol; 1 g fibre
Exchanges: 1/2 starch; 1 meat; 1/2 fat

BAKED WHOLE FISH WITH MINT VINAIGRETTE

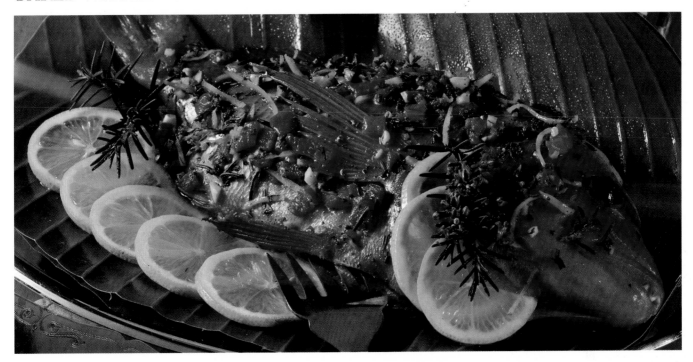

60 ml red wine vinegar
10 ml olive-oil
15 ml chopped fresh mint
10 ml finely chopped fresh rosemary
2 cloves of garlic, finely chopped
juice and shredded rind of half a lemon
half a small red pepper, seeded and diced *or*
    1 canned pimiento, chopped
3 ml salt
3 ml freshly ground black pepper
1 kg whole fresh white fish, e.g. Red Roman,
    Grunter, Stumpnose
lemon slices and fresh rosemary *or* mint sprigs
    to garnish

Combine first nine ingredients in a mixing-bowl. Cover and leave to stand one hour. Place fish on a large sheet of foil, lightly sprayed with non-stick spray. Make three diagonal cuts on both sides of fish, pour over herb mixture. Wrap in foil, securing well. Place on rack of roasting-pan, bake in 180 °C oven, or braai over glowing coals, about 30 minutes, or until fish flakes easily when tested with two forks. Transfer fish to suitable serving platter, drizzle herb mixture over fish. Garnish with lemon slices and fresh rosemary. Serve at once, with plain brown rice or a rice salad.

Serves four

Per serving: 872kJ; 1,2 g carbohydrate; 32,6 g protein; 7,2 g fat;
64 mg cholesterol; 0,2 g fibre
Exchanges: 4 meat

KEDGEREE

600 g frozen smoked haddock fillets, skinned
10 ml sunflower oil
1 onion, finely sliced
2 ml chilli-powder
5 ml turmeric
5 ml medium curry-powder
3 ml ground ginger
3 ml ground coriander
3 ml cumin seeds
2 ml ground mixed spice
5 ml salt *or* to taste
freshly ground black pepper to taste
400 g (500 ml) raw brown rice
25 ml finely chopped parsley
2 hard-boiled eggs, shelled and quartered (optional)

Poach haddock in water to cover, about 10 minutes, or until fish flakes easily when tested with two forks. Drain, reserve cooking liquid. Flake fish, remove any bones. Set fish aside, keep warm. Strain cooking liquid, measure 1,25 litres, adding extra water if necessary. Set aside. Heat oil in a large saucepan, add next 10 ingredients , sauté two minutes. Add rice, stir well, add reserved liquid. Bring to the boil, stir well, cover, reduce heat and cook over low heat until all the liquid has been absorbed, about 25 minutes. Stir rice with a fork, add fish and parsley. Cook a further five minutes, uncovered, or until thoroughly heated through. Transfer to a heated serving platter, garnish with hard-boiled egg wedges, serve at once.

Serves eight

Per serving: 862kJ; 22,1 g carbohydrate; 17,7 g protein; 3,9 g fat;
99 mg cholesterol; 2 g fibre
Exchanges: 1 1/2 starch; 2 meat

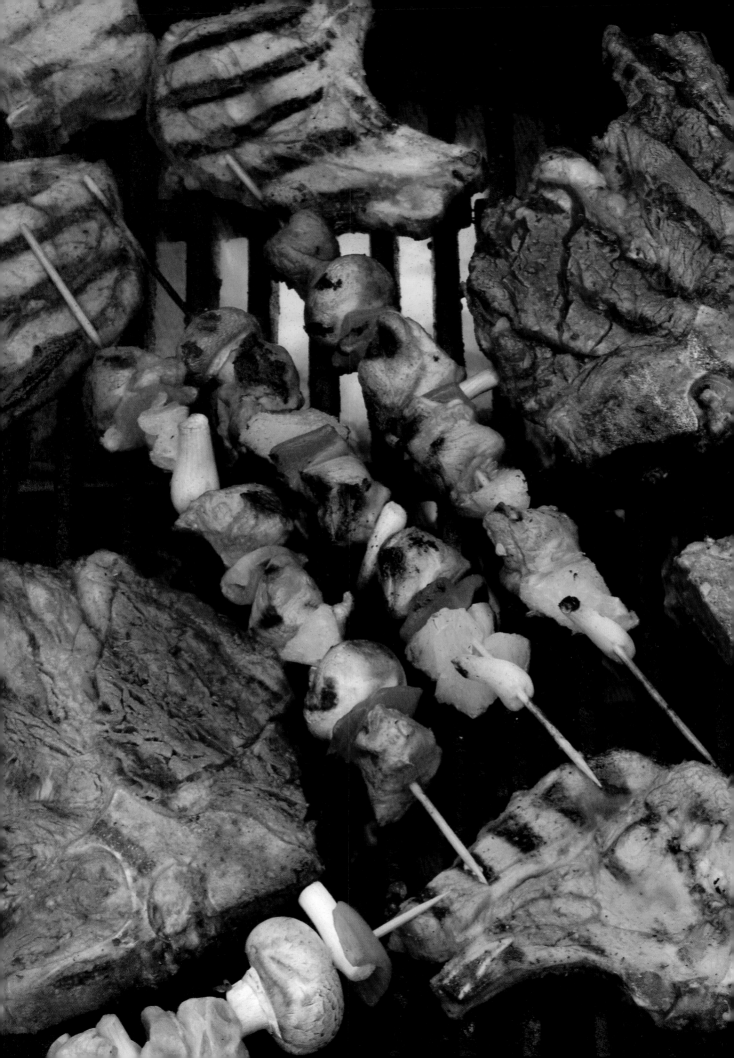

MEAT

This section includes beef, pork and lamb. Red meat, although a valuable source of protein, iron and Vitamin B_{12}, is high in cholesterol and should not be served more than two or three times a week. Keep to portions of 125 g raw meat per person, and trim off all visible fat. Use fat-free cooking methods wherever possible, and drain off any oil from the pan if frying or browning. Cheaper cuts, especially offal, are very high in fat and cholesterol, and have been omitted from this section.

INDIAN PORK CHOPS

1 fresh chilli, seeded and finely chopped
2 cloves of garlic, crushed
5 ml turmeric
5 ml dried coriander
5 ml cumin seeds
3 ml salt
1 ml whole black peppercorns
50 ml low-fat plain yoghurt
4 pork chops, trimmed of all fat

Crush first seven ingredients in a pestle and mortar into a paste. Stir into yoghurt. Spread over chops, cover and marinate 24 hours in refrigerator. Remove chops, wipe clean with absorbent kitchen paper towels. Grill on braai or under preheated griller, about seven minutes on each side, or until cooked through. Serve with baby potatoes and a cucumber salad.

Serves four

Per serving: 1 019kJ; 1,6 g carbohydrate; 26 g protein; 14 g fat; 87 mg cholesterol; 0,1 g fibre
Exchanges: 3 meat

LAMB KEBABS

Tea marinade
250 ml strong cold tea
1 clove of garlic, crushed
25 mm piece fresh ginger, peeled and grated
37,5 ml dry sherry
12,5 ml olive-oil

500 g lean lamb, trimmed of all fat and cut into
   25 mm cubes
16 large spring onions, green parts trimmed off
16 baby button mushrooms, wiped
2 red peppers, seeded and cut into large squares
2 oranges, thickly peeled and cut into segments

Combine all marinade ingredients, add lamb cubes. Cover and marinate overnight in refrigerator. Soak eight wooden skewers or satay sticks in water, 10 minutes, drain. Remove lamb cubes from marinade, reserve marinade. Thread drained lamb cubes, spring onion bulbs, mushrooms, peppers and orange segments alternately on to skewers. Grill on braai or under preheated griller, seven to eight minutes on each side, basting frequently with reserved marinade.

Serves four

Per serving: 1 074kJ; 13,5 g carbohydrate; 24,3 g protein; 9,4 g fat; 70 mg cholesterol; 3,7 g fibre
Exchanges: 2 vegetable; 1/2 fruit; 2 1/2 meat; 1/2 fat

MARINATED T-BONE STEAKS

Marinade
125 ml dry red wine
37,5 ml sunflower oil
90 ml water
25 ml soy sauce
1 ml liquid artificial sweetener
1 clove of garlic, crushed
3 ml ground ginger
3 ml dried origanum

4 T-bone steaks, trimmed of all fat

Combine all marinade ingredients in a glass or ceramic, shallow, rectangular dish. Arrange steaks in dish, turn to coat with marinade. Cover and refrigerate overnight. Drain steaks, reserve marinade. Grill on braai, or under preheated griller, basting occasionally with reserved marinade.

Serves four

Per serving: 1 517kJ; 1 g carbohydrate; 34,3 g protein; 21,5 g fat; 96 mg cholesterol; 0 g fibre
Exchanges: 4 meat; 2 fat

◄ Indian pork chops; Lamb kebabs; Marinated T-bone steaks

HOME-MADE BEEF STOCK

2 kg beef chuck bones
2 onions, quartered
2 celery stalks, chopped, including leaves
2 carrots, scraped and sliced
3 cloves of garlic, roughly chopped (optional)
10 whole black peppercorns
3 whole cloves
2 sprigs of thyme
2 bay-leaves

Exchanges: free

Step 1:

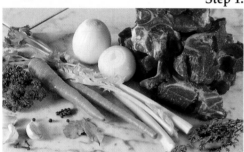

Collect all ingredients.

Step 2:

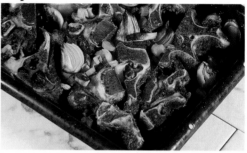

Place bones, onions, celery and carrots in a roasting-pan. Roast at 220 °C, one hour, or until well browned.

Step 3:

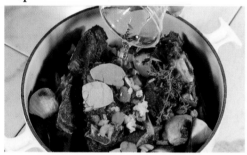

Transfer contents of roasting-pan to a large saucepan. Pour 500 ml boiling water into roasting-pan, scrape bottom of pan to loosen sediment, add to saucepan. Add remaining ingredients, cover with water. Bring to the boil. Reduce heat, cover and simmer gently three to four hours, skimming occasionally.

Step 4:

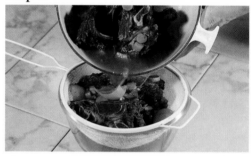

Strain stock through a fine sieve, discard contents of sieve. Allow stock to cool, refrigerate overnight.

Step 5:

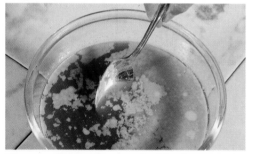

Remove layer of congealed fat from surface.

Step 6:

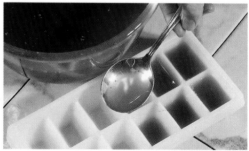

Cover bowl and store in refrigerator for two to three days, or spoon into ice-cube trays and freeze for up to six months.

Makes about three litres

26

MUSHROOM MEAT PATTIES

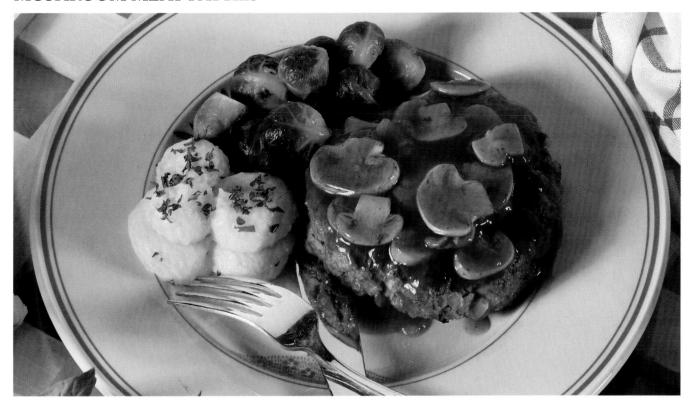

750 g lean beef mince
2 onions, finely chopped
125 ml cooked unsalted brown rice (35 g raw rice)
1 ml freshly ground black pepper
1 egg-white, lightly frothed
200 g button mushrooms, wiped and sliced
10 ml soy sauce
3 ml dried basil
750 ml home-made beef stock (see Pg 26)
10 g (25 ml) cornflour, mixed with
50 ml water

Place first five ingredients in a mixing-bowl, mix well
with hands. Form into eight patties, each about 20 mm
thick. Fry in non-stick frying-pan or electric frying-pan,
lightly sprayed with nonstick spray, five minutes on
each side, or until nicely browned. Remove and drain on
absorbent kitchen paper towels, set aside.

Wipe out pan, spray again with non-stick spray. Fry
mushrooms, three minutes, stirring continuously. Add
soy sauce, basil and stock, cook 10 minutes. Return
patties to pan, cover and cook slowly 10 to 15 minutes,
or until cooked through. Remove patties, transfer to a
heated serving dish, keep warm. Thicken gravy with
cornflour paste. Cook one to two minutes, stirring. Serve
patties topped with mushroom gravy, with Brussels
sprouts and mashed potato as accompaniments.

Serves eight

Per serving: 781kJ; 7,4 g carbohydrate; 20,1 g protein; 7,8 g fat; 61
mg cholesterol; 1,1 g fibre
Exchanges: 1/2 vegetable; 2 meat

SESAME PORK SCHNITZELS

8 pork escalopes
salt and freshly ground black pepper to taste
2 egg-whites, lightly frothed
120 g (250 ml) dry wholewheat breadcrumbs
100 g (165 ml) sesame seeds
5 ml olive-oil
lemon slices to garnish

Heat a baking tray in 220 °C oven while preparing
schnitzels. Pound escalopes with a meat mallet until
thin, sprinkle both sides with salt and pepper. Place egg-
whites in a shallow bowl. Combine crumbs and seeds,
place in a second bowl. Dip escalopes first into egg-
white, then into crumb mixture, coating well on both
sides. Brush olive-oil over surface of heated baking tray,
arrange escalopes on tray. Bake at 220 °C, five to six
minutes until crisp and golden brown. Turn and cook
the other side, a further four to five minutes, pressing
down firmly to keep them flat. Serve hot, garnished with
lemon slices, and with a mixed salad as accompaniment.

Serves four

Per serving: 2 963kJ; 31,4 g carbohydrate; 48,9 g protein; 43,6 g fat;
136 mg cholesterol; 2,8 g fibre
Exchanges: 1 starch; 5 1/2 meat; 3 fat

BEEF AND BEAN CASSEROLE

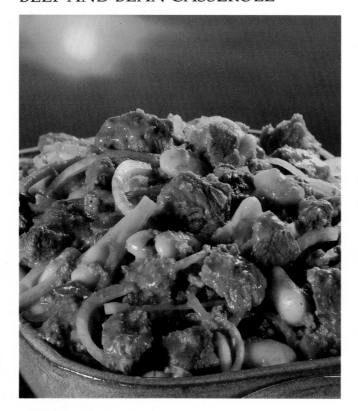

OATY BURGERS

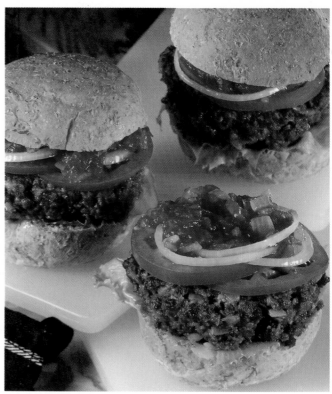

1 kg lean stewing steak
60 g (125 ml) wholewheat flour, seasoned with
10 ml salt and
5 ml freshly ground black pepper
15 ml olive-oil
3 carrots, scraped and cut julienne
2 onions, finely sliced into rings
7 ml ground mixed spice
2 bay-leaves
1 clove of garlic, crushed
1 red pepper, seeded and diced
1 green pepper, seeded and sliced into strips
1,2 litres home-made beef stock (see Pg 26)
450 g can lima *or* butter beans, drained

Trim all fat off meat, cut into 25 mm cubes. Coat in
seasoned flour, shake off excess. Heat 10 ml olive-oil in a
large saucepan, brown meat cubes, a few at a time,
remove with slotted spoon, drain on absorbent kitchen
paper towels. Heat remaining olive-oil in same pan, add
carrots, onions, spice, bay-leaves, garlic and peppers to
same pan, fry lightly, stirring well. Return meat cubes to
pan, add stock, bring to the boil, stirring all the time.
Reduce heat, cover and simmer one-and-a-half to two
hours, stirring occasionally, until meat is tender. Add
can of beans, cook a further five minutes or until heated
through. Remove bay-leaves. Serve with boiled potatoes
or brown rice, and a green vegetable.

Serves eight

Per serving: 1 343kJ; 16,3 g carbohydrate; 27,9 g protein; 13,1 g fat;
74 mg cholesterol; 6,2 g fibre
Exchanges: 1/2 vegetable; 1 starch; 2 1/2 meat; 1/2 fat

500 g lean beef mince
60 g (125 ml) rolled oats
1 onion, finely chopped
5 ml dried mixed herbs
salt and freshly ground black pepper to taste
6 lettuce leaves
6 wholewheat hamburger buns, split and spread
   with margarine
2 large ripe tomatoes, sliced
1 small onion, sliced and pushed into rings
Home-made tomato sauce (see Pg 90)

Combine mince, oats, onion, herbs and seasoning in a
small mixing-bowl, mix well with hands. Form mixture
into six patties, refrigerate one hour. Grill under
preheated griller, 15 to 20 minutes, turning once or
twice, until nicely browned and cooked through. Place a
lettuce leaf on half a bun, top with mince patty. Arrange
a few tomato slices and onion rings on patty, spoon a
little tomato sauce on top. Cover with second half of bun
and serve at once.

Serves six

Per serving: 1 427kJ; 38,2 g carbohydrate; 23,6 g protein; 9,6 g fat;
56 mg cholesterol; 6,5 g fibre
Exchanges: 1/2 vegetable; 2 starch; 2 meat; 2 fat

SWEET AND SOUR MEATBALLS

500 g lean beef mince
1 small onion, grated
85 g (350 ml) wholewheat
  breadcrumbs
salt and pepper to taste
1 small egg, beaten
300 ml home-made beef stock
  (see Pg 26)
1 celery stalk, washed and
  finely diced
1 carrot, scraped and diced
1 small ripe pineapple, peeled
  and finely diced
1 small leek, washed and
  finely sliced
50 ml brown vinegar
50 ml tomato purée
12,5 ml soy sauce
few drops of liquid artificial
  sweetener

Combine beef mince, onion,
crumbs, seasoning and egg in
a bowl. Mix well with hands.
Form into small balls. Set aside.
Place remaining ingredients,
except sweetener, in a
saucepan, bring to the boil.
Add meatballs, reduce heat,
cover and simmer 20 to
25 minutes, stirring
occasionally. Adjust seasoning
to taste, add sweetener.
Serve hot with ribbon noodles,
sprinkled with poppy or
sesame seeds, and broccoli.

Serves four

Per serving: 1 546kJ; 33,2 g
carbohydrate; 29,7 g protein; 12 g fat;
136 mg cholesterol; 4,1 g fibre
Exchanges: 1/2 vegetable; 1 fruit;
1 starch; 3 meat

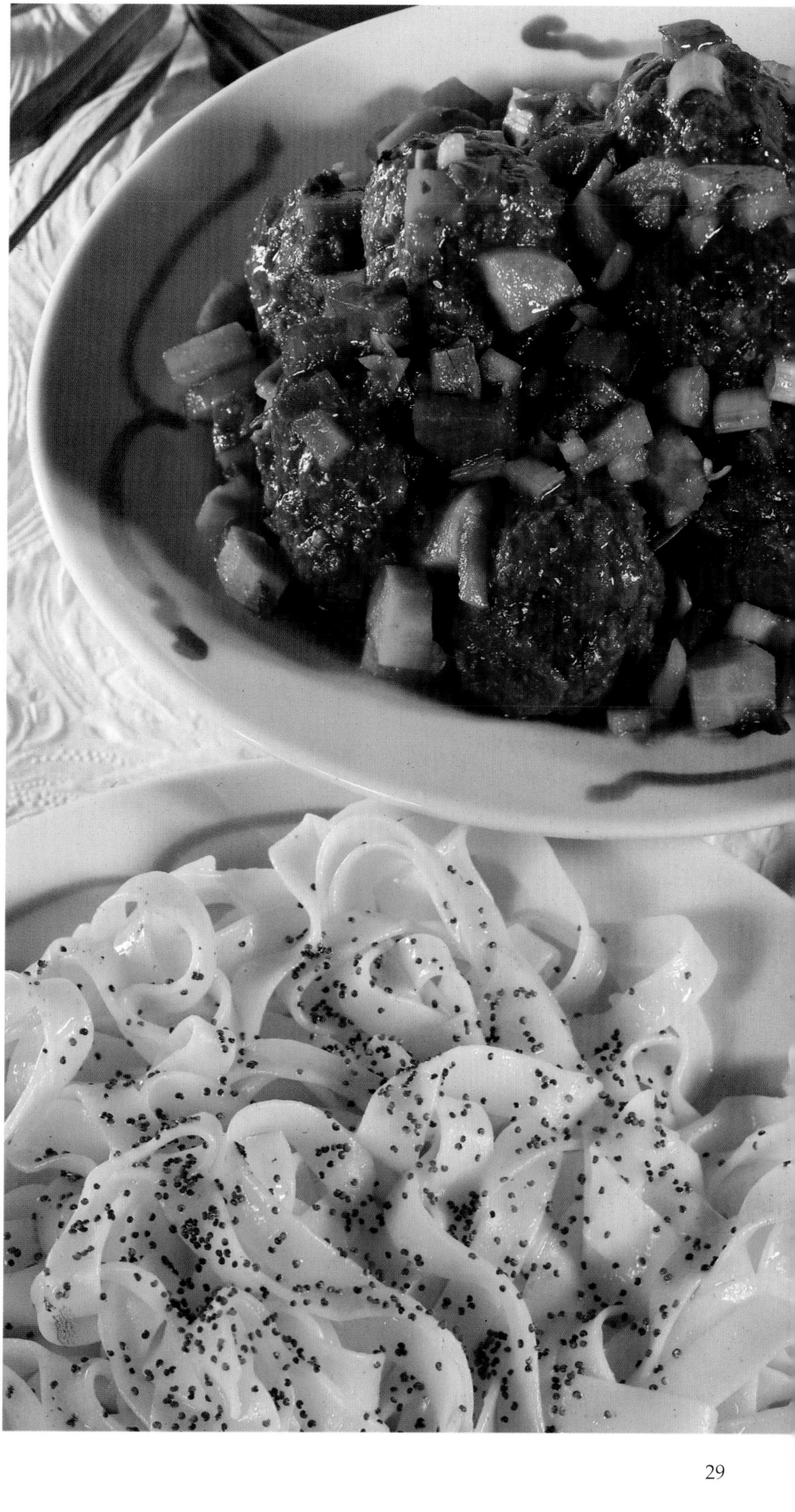

29

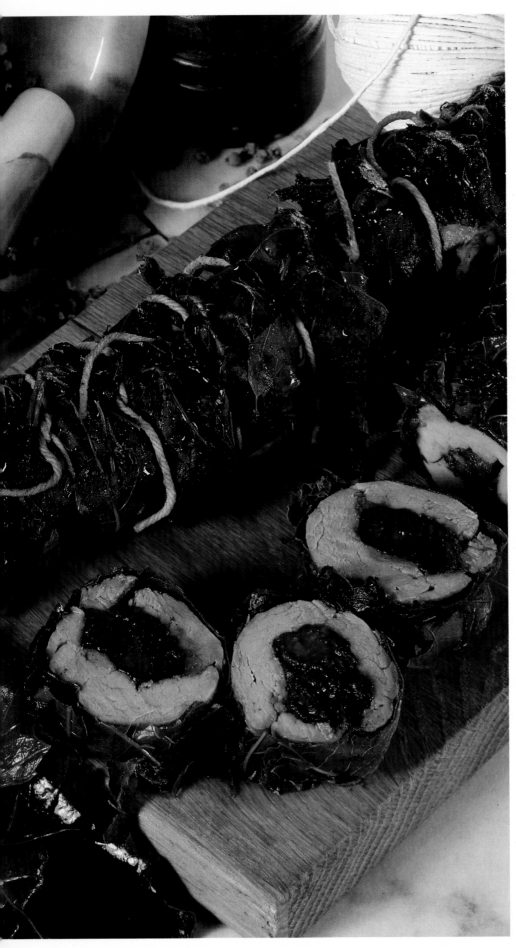

WRAPPED PORK WITH PRUNES

Cabbage, spinach or fresh grape leaves may be used instead of the vine leaves. Blanch in boiling water for a few minutes to soften before using.

200 g (330 ml) prunes
boiling water
25 ml brandy
juice and finely grated rind of
    one orange
2 pork fillets, about 400 g each,
    trimmed
salt and freshly ground black
    pepper to taste
200 g packet vine leaves in
    brine, well rinsed and
    drained
125 ml home-made chicken
    stock (see Pg 34)

Place prunes in a bowl, pour over enough boiling water to cover, add brandy, orange juice and rind. Cover and leave to soak at least four hours, or overnight. Drain, reserve liquid. Stone prunes. Flatten pork fillets by cutting lengthwise along one side, open out and beat with a meat mallet. Season lightly. Arrange prunes down centre of each fillet, roll up. Carefully wrap vine leaves around meat, tie at regular intervals with string. Place in roasting-pan, pour in stock. Cover pan with foil, shiny side inside, roast at 220 °C, 30 to 45 minutes, or until juices run clear. Remove from oven, allow to rest 10 minutes before carving. Add reserved prune liquid to contents of roasting-pan, bring to the boil. Boil until reduced by half, stirring and scraping. Strain into gravy boat. Remove string from meat, slice and arrange on heated serving platter. Serve gravy separately.

Serves six

Per serving: 1 736kJ; 21,4 g carbohydrate; 30,8 g protein; 20,9 g fat; 113 mg cholesterol; 2,4 g fibre
Exchanges: 1 1/2 fruit; 3 1/2 meat

30

PORK STIR-FRY

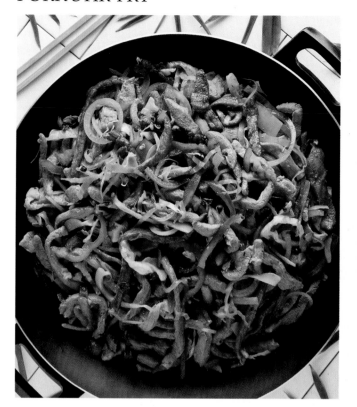

50 ml olive-oil
1 kg pork fillet, trimmed and cut into thin strips
3 celery stalks, sliced
2 green peppers, seeded and finely sliced
1 red pepper *or* canned pimiento, seeded and
  finely sliced
1 onion, thinly sliced into rings
100 g mushrooms, wiped and sliced
one-quarter small cabbage, finely shredded
12,5 ml soy sauce
salt and freshly ground black pepper to taste
100 g bean sprouts
230 g can sliced bamboo shoots, drained

Heat olive-oil in a large saucepan or wok, brown pork
strips a few at a time, over high heat. Remove and drain
on absorbent kitchen paper towels, set aside. Add next
six ingredients to same oil, stir-fry three to four minutes.
Stir in soy sauce and seasoning. Add sprouts and bamboo shoots , stir-fry until heated through and vegetables
are cooked but still crisp. Serve at once, with brown rice.

Serves eight

Per serving: 1 691kJ; 6 g carbohydrate; 30,3 g protein; 27,7 g fat;
106 mg cholesterol; 2,2 g fibre
Exchanges: 1 vegetable; 3 meat; 1 fat

ROAST LAMB WITH FRESH HERBS

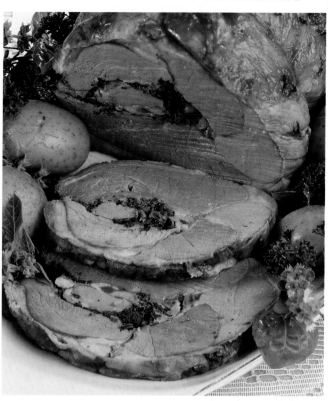

2 kg boned leg of lamb, trimmed of all fat
salt and freshly ground black pepper

Fresh herb stuffing
50 ml finely chopped parsley
25 ml chopped fresh mint
12,5 ml chopped fresh sage
10 ml chopped fresh thyme
10 ml chopped fresh rosemary
25 ml chopped fresh basil
2 cloves of garlic, crushed
10 ml freshly squeezed lemon juice
10 ml olive-oil
340 ml can dry apple cider

Rub meat on both sides with salt and pepper. Combine
all dry ingredients for stuffing, spread over meat, roll up
firmly, secure at regular intervals with string. Brush
lemon juice and olive-oil over roll, place in roasting-pan,
sprayed with non-stick spray. Roast at 200 °C,
20 minutes. Pour can of cider around meat, pour in an
equal can of water. Cover with foil, shiny side against
meat, and roast at 180 °C, one-and-a-half hours, basting
occasionally with liquid in pan. Remove meat from
roasting-pan, cover and keep warm. Boil liquid in pan
until well reduced, serve as gravy with the meat, with
assorted vegetables as accompaniments.

Serves eight

Per serving: 1 022kJ; 2,2 g carbohydrate; 32,1 g protein; 9,7 g fat;
101 mg cholesterol; 0 g fibre
Exchanges: 4 meat

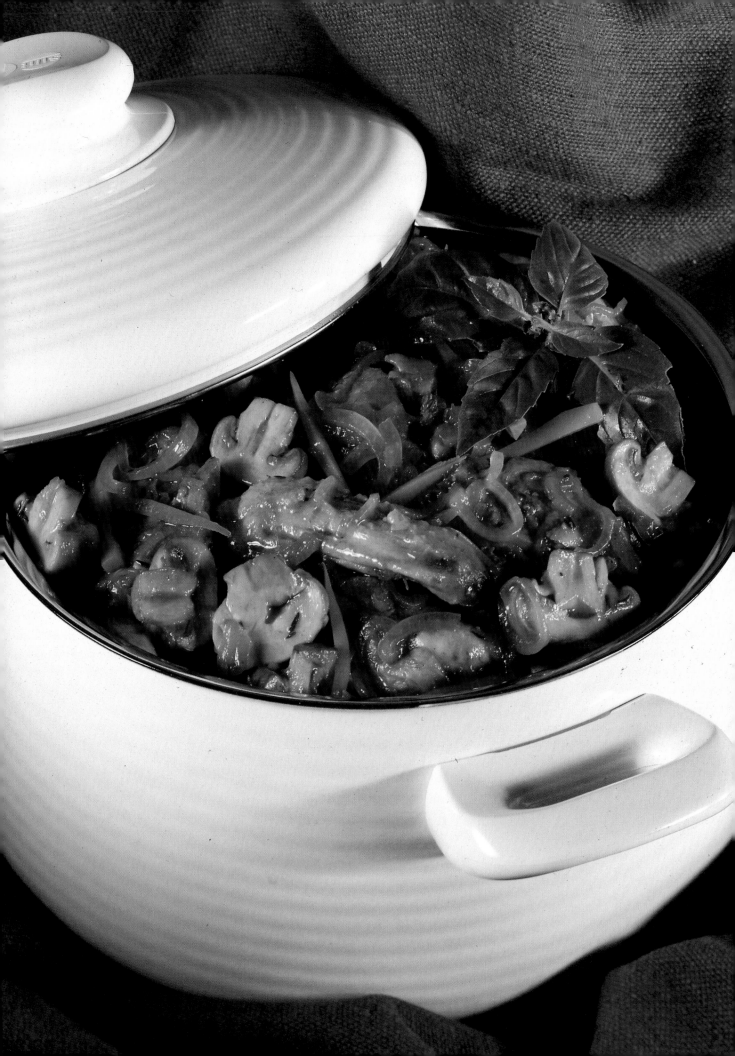

POULTRY

Although poultry embraces chickens, ducks, geese and turkeys, we've focussed mainly on chicken. It's the type most frequently eaten, economically priced, and freely available all year round. We have included duck recipes, too; but turkey has been allocated to the Special Occasions section. Of course, turkey and chicken meat are interchangeable, as are duck and goose; but remember to remove skin and all visible fat before preparing or serving, to reduce fat content and, therefore, kilojoules. Poultry is an excellent source of protein – it's lean, lower in kilojoules than red meat, and more easily digested. It can be presented in a myriad guises, its mild flavour blending well with sweet fruit, tangy cheese, or any number of herbs and spices. A 1,5 kg bird will feed six people, or about 90 g cooked meat per person.

COQ AU VIN

1,2 kg chicken pieces, skinned
37,5 ml olive-oil
2 large onions, thinly sliced
2 cloves of garlic, crushed
190 ml dry red wine *or* home-made chicken stock
   (see Pg 34)
60 ml brandy *or* unsweetened orange juice
250 ml home-made chicken stock
25 ml tomato paste
3 ml dried marjoram
2 ml pinch of herbs
3 ml salt
1 ml freshly ground black pepper
300 g small button mushrooms, left whole or halved
3 carrots, scraped and cut julienne
12 g (25 ml) cornflour, mixed to a paste with
50 ml water

Brown chicken pieces in heated olive-oil, half at a time. Remove and drain on absorbent kitchen paper towels, set aside. Fry onions and garlic in same pan, add wine, brandy, stock and tomato paste, stir well. Bring to the boil, add herbs and seasoning. Return chicken pieces to saucepan, add mushrooms and carrots. Cover, reduce heat, simmer 40 minutes. Remove chicken and vegetables, thicken gravy with cornflour paste. Cook two to three minutes, return chicken and vegetables, heat through. Serve hot, with baked potatoes and a green salad.

Serves six

Per serving: 1 763kJ; 21,4 g carbohydrate; 34,8 g protein; 15,8 g fat; 94 mg cholesterol; 2,5 g fibre
Exchanges: 1 vegetable; 3 1/2 meat; 1 fat

CHICKEN ASPARAGUS ROLLS

4 boneless chicken breast fillets
1 ml garlic salt
2 ml dried rosemary
3 ml salt
freshly ground black pepper to taste
60 g low-fat hard cheese, sliced
440 g can asparagus spears, drained
1 ml paprika
10 ml grated Parmesan cheese

Pound chicken fillets with a mallet until thin. Sprinkle with seasonings and herbs. Divide cheese slices between fillets, top with three or four asparagus spears each. Fold chicken fillet over asparagus, secure with toothpicks. Sprinkle with paprika, arrange, seam-side down, in a lightly greased, shallow ovenproof dish. Cover and bake at 180 °C, 30 minutes, or until chicken is tender. Carefully remove toothpicks, sprinkle with Parmesan cheese and serve at once, with baked potatoes and a mixed salad.

Serves four

Per serving: 840kJ; 3 g carbohydrate; 31,7 g protein; 6,2 g fat; 70 mg cholesterol; 1,7 g fibre
Exchanges: 1/2 vegetable; 3 meat

◀ *Coq au vin*

HOME-MADE CHICKEN STOCK

Use left-over chicken bones, skin, giblets and neck for an economical stock. If using a whole bird, strip off all flesh after about one hour's cooking, and keep for another use. Return carcass to stock pot and continue simmering a further one to two hours.

2 kg chicken *or* chicken bones and trimmings
2 large carrots, scraped and sliced
2 celery stalks, sliced
2 large onions, finely sliced
2 sprigs of thyme
2 bay-leaves
5 stems of parsley
8-10 black peppercorns

Exchanges: free

Step 1:

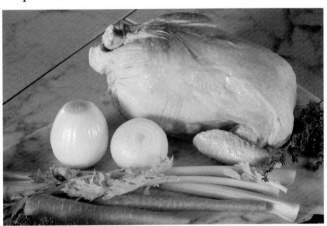

Collect all ingredients.

Step 2:

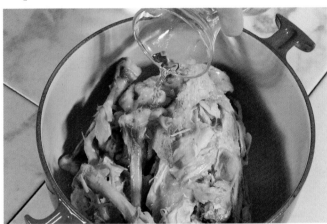

Place chicken, without giblets, in a large, heavy-bottomed saucepan. Pour in enough water to cover, bring to the boil. Boil 15 minutes, skim off any scum.

Step 3:

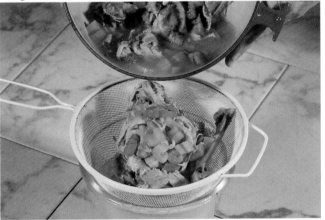

Add remaining ingredients, including giblets (except liver). Add more water to cover, return to the boil. Reduce heat, cover and simmer gently two to three hours. Strain stock through a fine sieve, discard contents of sieve. Cover stock, refrigerate overnight.

Step 4:

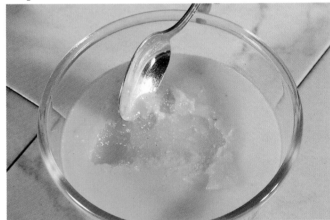

Remove congealed fat from surface. Cover stock, store in refrigerator three to four days, or transfer to suitable freezer containers or ice-cube trays and freeze for up to six months.

Makes about 2,5 litres

CHICKEN BREAST FILLETS WITH ROSEMARY

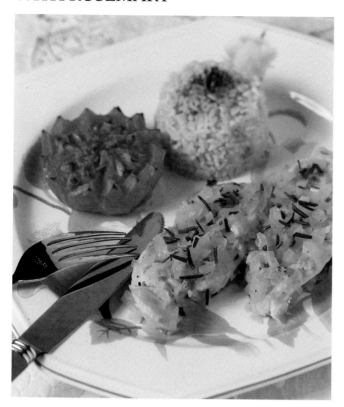

CHICKEN WITH ARTICHOKES AND POTATOES

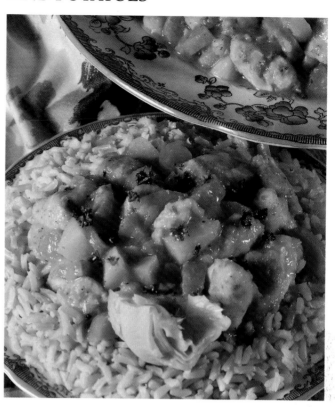

12,5 ml olive-oil
4 chicken breast fillets, skinned
2 cloves of garlic, crushed
12,5 ml chopped fresh rosemary *or* 5 ml dried rosemary
salt and freshly ground black pepper to taste
1 onion, finely chopped
125 ml dry white wine *or* home-made chicken stock
  (see Pg 34)
125 ml water

Heat olive-oil in non-stick frying-pan, brown chicken fillets with garlic. Stir in rosemary, seasoning and onion, fry two minutes. Stir in wine and water, bring to the boil. Cover, reduce heat, simmer 20 minutes. Remove chicken, place on four serving plates, cover and keep warm. Boil sauce until well reduced. Spoon over chicken. Serve with moulded brown rice and vandyked grilled tomato.

Serves four

600 g boned chicken pieces, skinned and cubed
wholewheat flour
salt and freshly ground black pepper to taste
25 ml olive-oil
1 large onion, finely chopped
2 cloves of garlic, crushed
300 ml home-made chicken stock (see Pg 34)
60 ml dry white wine *or* water
3 carrots, scraped and cubed
2 large potatoes, peeled and cubed
400 g can artichoke hearts in water, drained
2 ml dried origanum
12,5 ml finely chopped parsley

Coat chicken cubes in flour seasoned with salt and pepper, shake off excess. Brown cubes in heated olive-oil, stirring all the time. Remove chicken cubes, set aside. To same pan, add onion and garlic, sauté two minutes. Return chicken cubes to pan, pour in stock and wine. Add carrot and potato cubes, bring to the boil. Reduce heat, cover and simmer 25 minutes. Stir in artichoke hearts and origanum, heat through. Serve hot, on a bed of brown rice. Garnish with chopped parsley.

Serves four

Per serving: 782kJ; 2,8 g carbohydrate; 23,4 g protein; 6,3 g fat; 61 mg cholesterol; 0,5 g fibre
Exchanges: 2 1/2 meat; 1/2 fat

Per serving: 1 409kJ; 17,1 g carbohydrate; 32,3 g protein; 13,2 g fat; 87 mg cholesterol; 1,8 g fibre
Exchanges: 3 vegetable; 1/2 bread; 3 1/2 meat; 1 fat

CHICKEN AND PEA COBBLER

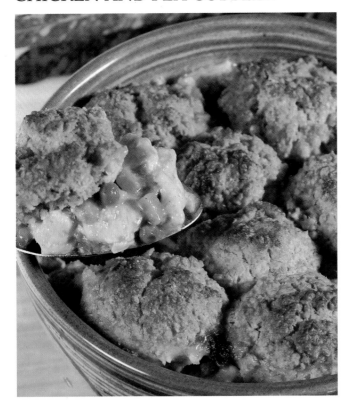

2 onions, finely chopped
2 carrots, scraped and diced
600 g frozen boneless chicken breast fillets, thawed
    and cubed
125 g margarine
30 ml dry sherry (optional)
325 ml home-made chicken stock (see Pg 34)
125 g (250 ml) wholewheat flour, sifted and husks
    replaced
5 ml chicken spice
3 ml salt
250 g frozen peas
70 g (190 ml) rolled oats
10 ml digestive bran
12,5 ml baking-powder
125 ml skim milk
1 egg-white, lightly frothed

Fry onions, carrots and chicken cubes in 25 g margarine,
10 minutes. Add sherry, if used, stock, 30 g (60 ml) flour,
spice and salt, cook three minutes, stirring all the time,
until thickened. Add peas, transfer to a lightly greased
1,5-litre ovenproof casserole dish. Combine remaining
flour, oats, bran and baking-powder in a mixing-bowl,
rub in remaining margarine until mixture resembles fine
crumbs. Stir in milk and egg-white to form a soft dough.
Drop about 60 ml amounts on to chicken mixture, bake
at 220 °C, 45 minutes or until well risen and golden
brown. Serve as a meal-in-one.

Serves six

Per serving: 1 952kJ; 29,6 g carbohydrate; 6,9 g protein; 23,6 g fat;
58 mg cholesterol; 6,5 g fibre
Exchanges: 1 vegetable; 1 starch; 2 1/2 meat; 4 fat

PRUNE AND DUCK CASSEROLE

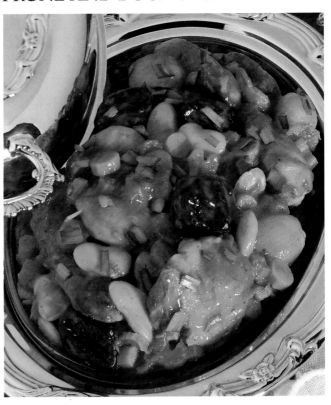

250 ml brandy *or* unsweetened orange juice
125 g prunes
200 g dried lima beans
25 ml olive-oil
2,2 kg duck, cut into serving portions, skin and fat
    removed
250 g baby pickling onions, peeled
12,5 ml wholewheat flour
1 carrot, scraped and sliced
1 celery stalk, sliced
5 ml dry mustard powder
3 bay-leaves
4 whole cloves
410 g can whole peeled tomatoes, undrained, chopped
250 ml home-made chicken stock (see Pg 34)
salt and pepper to taste
chopped chives to garnish

Pour brandy over prunes in a small mixing-bowl, cover
and leave to macerate overnight. Cover beans with
water, leave to soak overnight. Heat olive-oil in a large
saucepan, fry duck pieces until brown, turning
frequently. Remove with slotted spoon, drain on
absorbent kitchen paper towels, transfer to lightly
greased ovenproof casserole dish, set aside. Add onions
to same saucepan, brown well on all sides. Stir in flour,
cook one minute. Add next seven ingredients, stir well,
bring to the boil. Remove prunes from brandy, stone,
add to saucepan with brandy and drained beans. Add
onion mixture to duck in casserole dish, cover and bake
at 180 °C, one hour. Discard bay-leaves and whole
cloves before serving. Garnish with chopped chives,
serve with brown rice and a green vegetable.

Serves four

ROAST DUCK WITH PEAR STUFFING

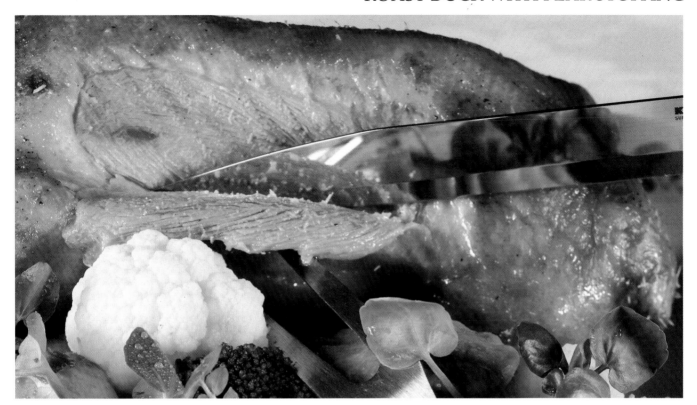

Skin is left on during roasting to prevent duck from drying out excessively. Remember to discard when carving.

**2,5 kg - 3 kg duck, washed, dried and any visible fat
  removed
water for steaming
10 ml olive-oil
4 cloves of garlic, crushed
500 g fresh pears, peeled, cored and finely diced
juice of one lemon
5 ml dried rosemary
salt and freshly ground black pepper**

Prick duck all over with a skewer or toothpick, place on rack of roasting-pan. Fill base of pan with water, cover completely with foil, shiny side inside. Steam at 190 °C, 30 minutes, to release fat. Heat olive-oil in a frying-pan, sauté garlic, one minute. Add remaining ingredients, cover and simmer gently 15 minutes. Set aside. Remove duck from oven, season well. Discard water. Stuff duck cavity with pear mixture, truss. Place on rack of roasting-pan, roast, uncovered, at 190 °C, one-and-a-half hours, or until juices run clear when pierced with a skewer. Do not overcook or duck will be tough and dry. Place duck on heated serving platter, garnish with dried pears and watercress. Serve with broccoli, cauliflower, baby patty pans and a thin gravy made from chicken stock and gravy browning.

Serves four

Prune and Duck Casserole
Per serving: 2 819kJ; 58,2 g carbohydrate; 58,2 g protein; 19,5 g fat; 152 mg cholesterol; 11,5 g fibre
Exchanges: 2 vegetable; 3 fruit; 2 starch; 4 1/2 meat; 1 fat

Per serving: 1 743kJ; 16,7 g carbohydrate; 48,6 g protein; 15,3 g fat; 146 mg cholesterol; 3,3 g fibre
Exchanges: 1 fruit; 4 1/2 meat; 1/2 fat

37

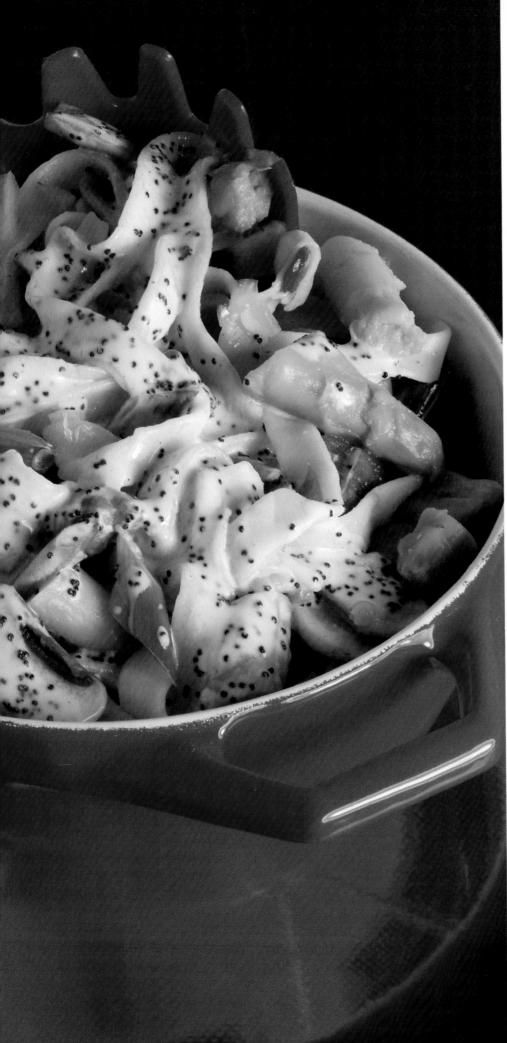

EGG NOODLES WITH ASPARAGUS AND POPPY SEEDS

250 g ribbon noodles
12,5 ml cooking oil
1 large onion, chopped
12,5 ml olive-oil
2 cloves of garlic, crushed
200 g button mushrooms,
  wiped and sliced
pinch of cayenne pepper
440 g can asparagus spears,
  drained and diagonally
  sliced
bunch of spring onions,
  trimmed and diagonally
  sliced
125 ml low-fat plain yoghurt
12,5 ml poppy seeds
salt and freshly ground black
  pepper to taste

Cook noodles in rapidly boiling
salted water with oil, until just
tender, 12 to 15 minutes. Drain
well, set aside. Sauté onion in
olive-oil in a saucepan, two
minutes. Add garlic, mushrooms and cayenne pepper,
sauté five minutes over high
heat. Reduce heat, stir in
asparagus, spring onions and
noodles, toss well.
Combine yoghurt, poppy seeds
and seasoning, pour over
noodle mixture, stir well to heat
through. Serve at once.

Serves six

Per serving: 952kJ; 28,8 g
carbohydrate; 9,4 g protein; 7,1 g fat;
32 mg cholesterol; 4,4 g fibre
Exchanges: 1 1/2 vegetable;
1 1/2 starch; 1 fat

RICE AND PASTA

These grain products add carbohydrate and some protein to the daily diet. If unrefined or enriched, they are excellent sources of vitamins and fibre. Besides providing energy and a long-lasting feeling of satisfaction after a meal, they are relatively low in kilojoules: 150 g cooked spaghetti contains only 840 kJ – half that of red meat. Although their protein is incomplete, a well-chosen sauce or an additional ingredient will provide the missing amino acids, making a complete meal. Economical to buy, rice and pasta lend themselves to an infinite variety of dishes. Both should feature regularly on the weekly menu .

CHICKEN AND RICE RING

Filling
75 ml home-made diabetic mayonnaise (see Pg 93)
3 ml medium curry-powder
30 g (50 ml) unsalted cashew nuts, chopped
200 g cooked chicken meat, cubed
salt and pepper to taste

Rice ring
240 g (300 ml) raw brown rice, cooked
200 g frozen mixed vegetables, cooked
25 ml cooking oil
12,5 ml white wine vinegar
1 ml dry mustard powder
1 ml paprika
chopped parsley to garnish

Filling
Combine all ingredients, season to taste. Set aside.

Rice ring
Combine rice with vegetables in a bowl. Whisk together oil, vinegar, mustard and paprika, add to rice mixture, toss well. Press into a lightly greased 200 mm-diameter ring mould. Smooth surface with the back of a spoon. Carefully turn out mould on to a flat plate. Spoon chicken mixture into centre. Serve chilled, garnished with chopped parsley.

Serves eight

Per serving: 737kJ; 16,4 g carbohydrate; 9,7 g protein; 7,1 g fat;
21 mg cholesterol; 2,2 g fibre
Exchanges: 1/2 vegetable; 1 starch; 1 meat; 1 fat

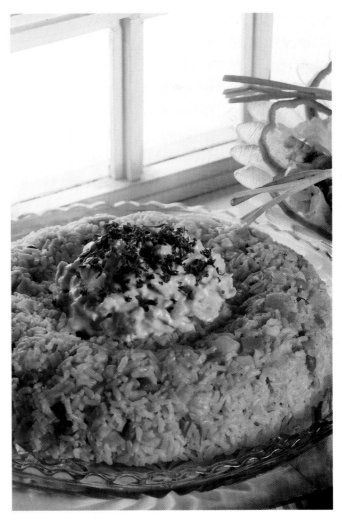

HAKE WITH PASTA SHELLS

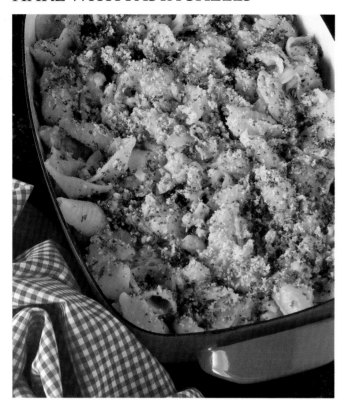

BRINJAL AND RICE BAKE

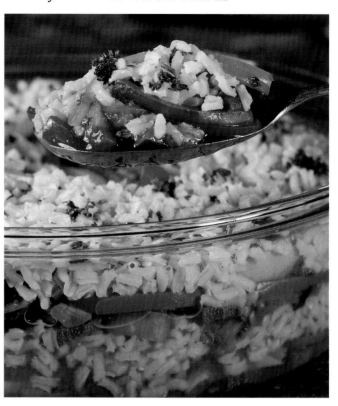

250 g pasta shells
12,5 ml cooking oil
10 ml olive-oil
1 onion, finely chopped
12 g (25 ml) wholewheat flour
350 ml home-made chicken *or* fish stock
   (see Pgs 34 and 20)
pinch of ground nutmeg
salt and freshly ground black pepper to taste
300 g hake fillets, skinned, cooked and flaked
12 g (50 ml) fresh brown breadcrumbs
6 g (15 ml) grated Parmesan cheese
paprika and chopped parsley to garnish

Cook pasta in rapidly boiling salted water with cooking oil, until just tender, 12 to 15 minutes. Drain well, set aside. Heat olive-oil in a saucepan, sauté onion two minutes. Stir in flour, cook one minute, stirring. Stir in stock, nutmeg and seasoning, bring to the boil, stirring continuously. Cook two minutes. Combine pasta and hake, stir into sauce. Transfer to a shallow, lightly greased ovenproof dish, top with breadcrumbs and cheese. Place under preheated griller until crumbs are crisp and golden brown. Sprinkle with paprika and chopped parsley before serving.

Serves six

10 ml olive-oil
3 cloves of garlic, crushed
2 large onions, sliced
1 large brinjal, cut into 10 mm cubes
3 baby marrows, thinly sliced
1 red pepper, seeded and cut into thin strips
1 green pepper, seeded and cut into thin strips
1 yellow pepper, seeded and cut into thin strips
410 g can whole peeled tomatoes, undrained and
   chopped
500 ml cooked brown rice (130 g raw)
salt and freshly ground black pepper to taste
60 ml home-made vegetable *or* chicken stock
   (see Pgs 44 and 34)
12,5 ml finely chopped parsley

Heat olive-oil in a saucepan, sauté garlic and onions three to four minutes. Cover and allow to sweat, two minutes. Add brinjal cubes and marrows, cover and cook slowly 15 minutes, stirring frequently. Set two-thirds of vegetable mixture aside. Spread remaining third in base of a lightly greased 1, 5-litre ovenproof dish. Add alternate layers of pepper strips, tomatoes, rice, reserved vegetable mixture and seasoning, until all ingredients are used up. Pour stock over casserole, sprinkle with parsley. Cover and bake at 180 °C, one hour, or until vegetables are very tender but not mushy. Serve at once.

Serves six as a main meal, or eight as a vegetable accompaniment.

Per serving: 1 109kJ; 30,6 g carbohydrate; 17,2 g protein; 6,8 g fat;
23 mg cholesterol; 2,1 g fibre
Exchanges: 1 1/2 starch; 1 1/2 meat; 1 fat

Per serving: 691kJ; 26,8 g carbohydrate; 4,4 g protein; 3,1 g fat; 0 mg
cholesterol; 4,8 g fibre
Exchanges: 2 vegetable; 1 1/2 starch

TWISTED PASTA WITH LENTILS

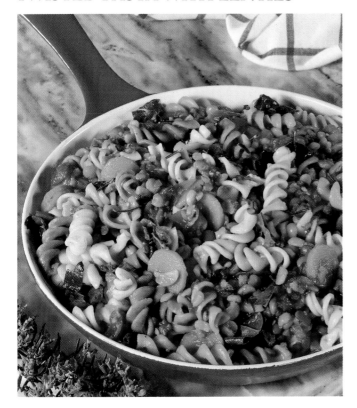

10 ml olive-oil
1 large onion, finely chopped
1 large carrot, scraped and sliced
4 cloves of garlic, crushed
500 ml home-made chicken stock (see Pg 34)
100 g (125 ml) lentils, rinsed
100 g (125 ml) split peas, rinsed
5 ml finely chopped fresh rosemary *or* 1 ml dried
   rosemary
10 ml finely chopped parsley
410 g can whole peeled tomatoes, undrained, chopped
200 g fresh spinach leaves, torn into bite-sized pieces
salt and freshly ground black pepper to taste
500 g twisted pasta shapes (*fusilli*)
12,5 ml cooking oil
4 g (10 ml) grated Parmesan cheese (optional)

Heat olive-oil in a large frying-pan, fry onion, carrot and garlic, three minutes. Add stock, lentils, peas, rosemary and parsley, bring to the boil. Reduce heat, cover and simmer 15 minutes. Add can of tomatoes with liquid, cover and simmer a further 15 minutes. Stir in spinach, cook until just wilted, about five minutes.
Season well, set aside. Cook pasta in rapidly boiling salted water with cooking oil, until just tender, about 12 minutes. Drain well, add to spinach mixture. Toss well over medium heat until heated through. Serve at once as a meal on its own, sprinkled with Parmesan cheese if desired.

Serves eight

Per serving: 1 492kJ; 54,7 g carbohydrate; 15,7 g protein; 5 g fat;
1 mg cholesterol; 8,6 g fibre
Exchanges: 1 vegetable; 3 starch; 1/2 fat

VEGETARIAN JAMBALAYA

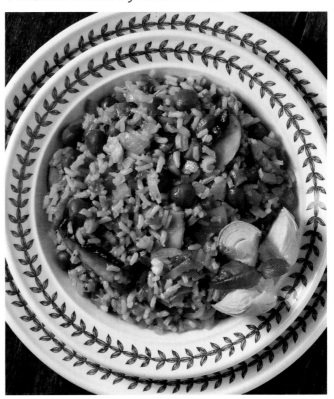

2 green peppers, seeded and diced
3 celery stalks, finely chopped
3 onions, finely chopped
4 cloves of garlic, crushed
410 g can whole peeled tomatoes, undrained, chopped
5 ml each freshly ground black pepper and salt
3 ml Tabasco sauce
5 ml dried sweet basil
5 ml dried thyme
3 bay-leaves
400 g (500 ml) raw brown rice
10 ml olive-oil
200 g large brown mushrooms, wiped and thinly sliced
410 g can dun peas, drained
400 g can artichoke hearts
cayenne pepper to sprinkle
fresh basil leaves to garnish (optional)

Place first 12 ingredients in a large saucepan. Add one litre water, cover, bring to the boil. Reduce heat, simmer 30 to 40 minutes, until all liquid has been absorbed and rice is tender. Discard bay-leaves. Heat olive-oil in a frying-pan, sauté mushrooms five minutes. Remove with slotted spoon. Add to rice mixture, together with dun peas, mix in gently. Place artichoke hearts in a small saucepan, bring to the boil. Drain and keep warm.
Pile on to a serving plate, and sprinkle with cayenne pepper. Garnish with artichoke wedges and fresh basil.

Serves eight

Per serving: 1 006kJ; 39,5 g carbohydrate; 8,9 g protein; 2,8 g fat;
0 mg cholesterol; 8,6 g fibre
Exchanges: 3 vegetable; 1 1/2 starch

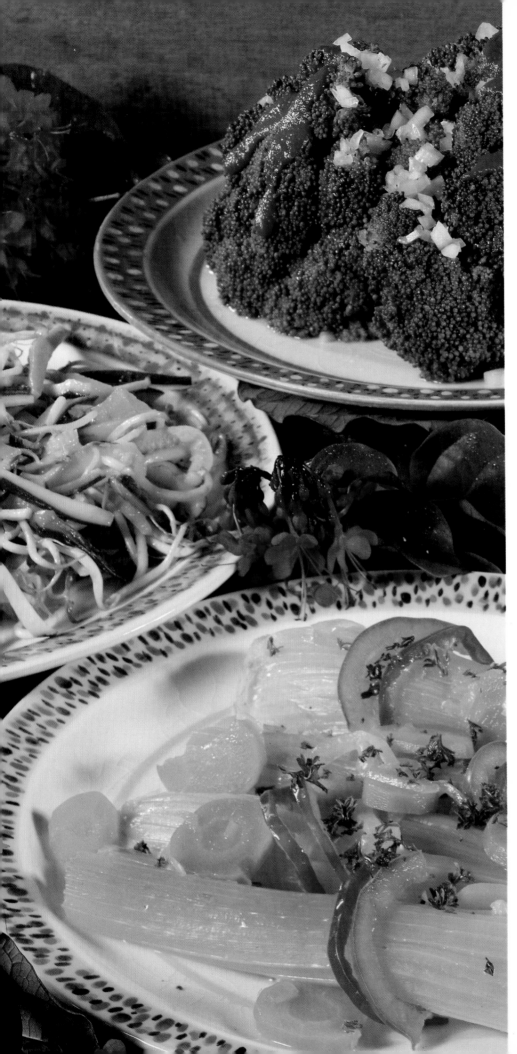

BEAN SPROUT STIR-FRY

20 ml sunflower oil
250 g baby marrows, trimmed
  and cut julienne
1 large carrot, scraped and cut
  julienne
3 spring onions, trimmed to
  70 mm lengths
salt and freshly ground black
  pepper to taste
125 g bean sprouts
12,5 ml dry sherry

Heat oil in a large frying-pan or
wok. Add baby marrows and
carrot, stir-fry one to two
minutes. Add spring onions,
stir-fry a further two to three
minutes. Season well, add bean
sprouts and sherry, toss well to
heat through. Serve at once.

Serves four to six

Per serving: 190kJ; 2,3 g carbohydrate;
1,3 g protein; 3 g fat; 0 mg cholesterol;
1,3 g fibre
Exchanges: 1 vegetable; 1 fat

Clockwise from top: Spicy broccoli
with puréed pepper; Braised celery
with peppers; Bean sprout stir-fry

VEGETABLES

They provide colour, texture and flavour to the menu, while contributing abundantly to our daily vitamin and mineral intake, Vitamins A and C in particular. Consisting of 70% to 90% water, vegetables are very low in kilojoules, cholesterol-free, low in sodium, and high in dietary fibre – good news for anyone wanting to follow a healthy lifestyle. Serve vegetables raw and freshly prepared as often as possible, to glean maximum nutritional value; or prepare them in any of the following tasty ways as a light main meal or colourful accompaniment.

SPICY BROCCOLI WITH PURÉED PEPPER

500 g head of broccoli, hard stalks trimmed
10 ml olive-oil
1 small onion, finely chopped and blanched one
 minute (reserve 10 ml)
2 cloves of garlic, crushed
3 red peppers *or* canned pimientos, seeded and diced
25 ml tomato purée
125 ml home-made vegetable stock (see Pg 44)
5 ml white wine vinegar
5 ml dried tarragon
5 ml prepared horse-radish sauce
salt and freshly ground black pepper to taste
few drops of liquid artificial sweetener (optional)

Steam broccoli over a saucepan of simmering water, about 25 minutes, or place, with 37,5 ml water, in a plastic bag, pierce bag, and microwave on 100% (High) power, about 10 minutes, or until stalks can be easily pierced with a wooden toothpick. Set aside, keep warm. Meanwhile, heat olive-oil in a frying-pan, sauté onion and garlic, two minutes. Add peppers, cook, stirring, until softened, two to three minutes. Add remaining ingredients, bring to the boil. Remove from heat, pour into food processor bowl, blend until smooth. Adjust seasoning to taste, add sweetener if desired. Transfer broccoli to a heated serving plate or vegetable bowl, spoon sauce over broccoli. Sprinkle with reserved chopped onion and serve at once.

Serves four to six

Per serving: 277kJ; 6,7 g carbohydrate; 3,4 g protein; 2,4 g fat; 0 mg cholesterol; 3,6 g fibre
Exchanges: 2 vegetable; 1/2 fat

BRAISED CELERY WITH PEPPERS

4 heads of celery
1 red pepper, seeded and thinly sliced into rings
1 green pepper, seeded and thinly sliced into rings
3 large carrots, scraped and thinly sliced
1 large onion, finely chopped
750 ml home-made vegetable *or* chicken stock
 (see Pgs 44 and 34)
salt and freshly ground black pepper to taste
1 ml cayenne pepper
5 ml dried mixed herbs
12,5 ml finely chopped parsley to garnish

Trim celery heads down to about 150 mm, keep leaves for stock or soup. Split each head in half, wash well under cold, running water, keeping stalks intact. Arrange neatly in a large, shallow saucepan. Cut pepper rings in half, scatter over celery. Add carrots, onion, stock, seasonings and mixed herbs, bring to the boil. Reduce heat, cover and simmer gently until celery is tender, about one-and-a-half hours. Carefully remove celery, arrange on a heated serving platter with carrots and peppers. Cover, keep warm. Boil stock left in saucepan until well reduced, spoon over celery before serving. Garnish with parsley.

Serves eight

Per serving: 85kJ; 3,5 g carbohydrate; 0,6 g protein; 0 g fat; 0 mg cholesterol; 1,1 g fibre
Exchanges: 1 vegetable

HOME-MADE VEGETABLE STOCK

For a truly economical stock, save water from cooking vegetables, plus any trimmings and peelings. Boil until well reduced, strain and store in refrigerator or freezer.

Exchanges: free

4 celery stalks, roughly chopped, including leaves
4 carrots, scraped and roughly chopped
4 large onions, roughly chopped
1 head of broccoli, roughly chopped
1 turnip, peeled and diced
4 cloves of garlic, peeled (optional)
1 bunch of parsley
6 black peppercorns
2 sprigs of thyme
3 bay-leaves

Step 1:

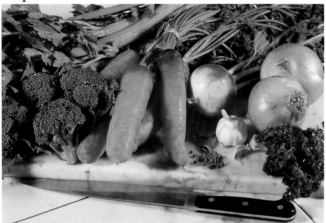

Collect all ingredients.

Step 2:

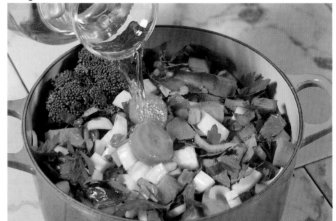

Place all ingredients in a large, heavy-bottomed saucepan, pour in enough water to cover. Bring to the boil. Reduce heat, cover and simmer one hour.

Step 3:

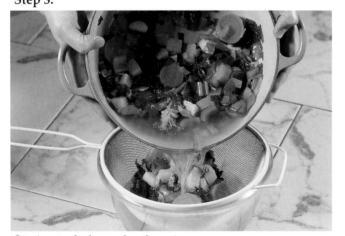

Strain stock through a fine sieve.

Step 4:

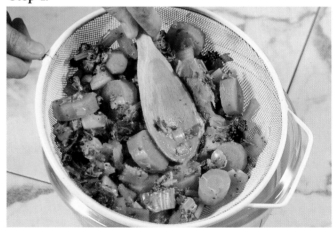

Press down firmly on vegetables in sieve, with the back of a wooden spoon, to extract as much liquid as possible. Discard contents of sieve. Allow stock to cool completely. Cover and store in refrigerator for up to one week, or pour into suitable freezer containers or ice-cube trays, and freeze for up to six months.

Makes about two litres

CURRIED MIXED VEGETABLES

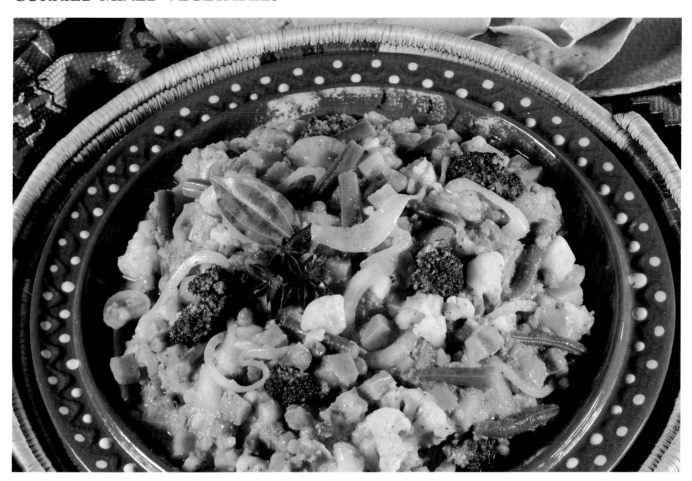

When serving as a main dish, add two or three chopped fresh chillies or extra chilli-powder, if desired. Serve with curry sambals and a home-made chutney.

2 large potatoes, peeled and cubed
250 g cauliflower, broken into florets
250 g broccoli, broken into florets
250 g carrots, scraped and diced
250 g green beans, topped, tailed and cut into
   50 mm lengths
125 g frozen peas, thawed
12,5 ml olive-oil
12,5 ml mustard seeds
5 ml cumin seeds
3 ml fenugreek
2 star anise
1 bay-leaf
5 ml turmeric
2 onions, thinly sliced
salt and freshly ground black pepper to taste
1 ml chilli-powder *or* to taste
60 ml water
2 large tomatoes, skinned and chopped
juice of half a lemon

Bring a saucepan of water to the boil. Blanch potato cubes, two minutes. Add cauliflower, broccoli and carrots, blanch three minutes. Add beans, blanch two minutes. Add peas, remove from heat immediately. Drain vegetables, rinse under cold, running water, set aside. Heat olive-oil in a large saucepan. Fry spices and onions, stirring all the time, two to three minutes. Add vegetables, salt, pepper, chilli-powder and water. Cover, cook gently five minutes. Add tomatoes and lemon juice, cook a further one minute. Adjust seasoning to taste, serve hot as a vegetable accompaniment to any plain meat or poultry dish, or as a vegetarian main course.

Serves six to eight

Per serving: 696kJ; 24,8 g carbohydrate; 6,6 g protein; 3,5 g fat; 0 mg cholesterol; 7,1 g fibre
Exchanges: 2 vegetable; 1/2 starch; 1/2 fat

PUMPKIN SOUFFLÉ

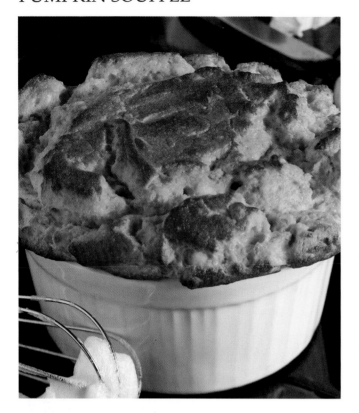

1 kg piece of pumpkin, seeded
40 g margarine
12 g (25 ml) dry breadcrumbs
12 g (25 ml) wholewheat flour
150 ml skim milk
2 egg-yolks
2 ml salt
1 ml freshly ground black pepper
5 ml ground cinnamon
10 g (25 ml) grated Parmesan cheese
4 egg-whites

Wrap pumpkin in sheet of foil, shiny side inside, place on baking tray. Bake at 200 °C, one-and-a-half hours, or until tender. Uncover, allow to cool. Remove skin, purée pumpkin pulp in electric blender or food processor. Turn into a saucepan, cook over medium heat until no longer wet, stirring all the time. Using 10 g margarine, grease inside of a 900 ml soufflé dish, sprinkle with breadcrumbs, shake out excess. Set aside.
Melt remaining margarine in a small saucepan, stir in flour, cook one minute. Add milk, cook, stirring continuously, until sauce is thick and smooth, remove from heat. Beat in egg-yolks one at a time, add seasoning, cinnamon and half the Parmesan cheese. Beat in the pumpkin purée. Whip egg-whites until soft peaks form, fold into pumpkin mixture. Turn mixture into prepared soufflé dish, sprinkle remaining Parmesan cheese over top. Bake at 190 °C, about 45 minutes, until well risen and firm. Serve immediately.

Serves six

Per serving: 805kJ; 14,7 g carbohydrate; 7,6 g protein; 10,4 g fat; 127 mg cholesterol; 5,1 g fibre
Exchanges: 1 starch; 1/2 meat; 1 1/2 fat

VEGETABLE HOT-POT

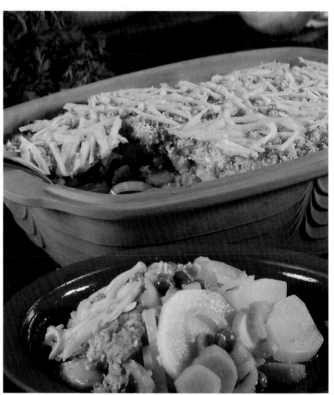

500 g carrots, scraped and thinly sliced
2 large onions, thinly sliced
3 celery stalks, trimmed and thinly sliced
500 g potatoes, peeled and thinly sliced
1 turnip, peeled and thinly sliced
500 ml home-made vegetable *or* chicken stock
  (see Pgs 44 and 34)
1 bouquet garni
salt and freshly ground black pepper to taste
425 g can butter beans, drained
125 g frozen peas
180 g (750 ml) fresh brown breadcrumbs
90 g (225 ml) low-fat hard cheese, grated

Layer carrots, onions, celery, potatoes and turnip in a 2,5-litre ovenproof casserole dish. Pour stock over vegetables, add bouquet garni and seasoning. Cover and bake at 180 °C, one-and-a-half hours. Remove and discard bouquet garni. Add butter beans and peas. Combine crumbs and grated cheese, sprinkle over casserole. Return to oven, uncovered, bake a further 30 to 40 minutes. Serve hot, as a delicious meal-in-one, with crusty wholewheat bread and a glass of dry cider.

Serves six to eight

(Based on six servings) Per serving: 1 664kJ; 61,3 g carbohydrate; 19,5 g protein; 1 g fat; 0 mg cholesterol; 19,4 g fibre
Exchanges: 1 vegetable; 2 1/2 starch; 1/2 meat

STUFFED PEPPERS

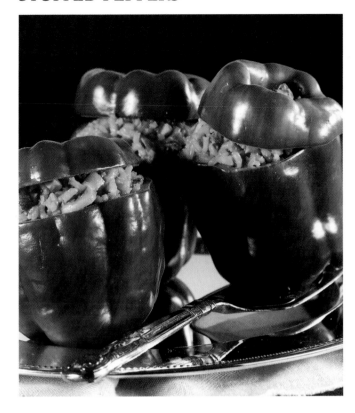

Stuff any variety of vegetables in the same way. Instead of rice, use cooked samp, canned corn, breadcrumbs, or left-over meat and vegetables for the filling.

4 large red *or* green peppers
25 g margarine
1 onion, finely chopped
150 g (190 ml) raw brown rice
25 ml tomato purée
500 ml home-made vegetable *or* chicken stock
  (see Pgs 44 and 34)
150 g button mushrooms, wiped and sliced
salt and freshly ground black pepper to taste
50 g (125 ml) hazel-nuts, chopped
10 ml soy sauce

Step 1:

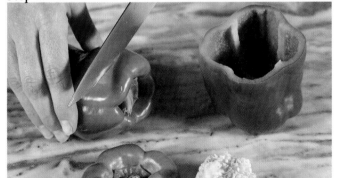

Cut a 25 mm lid off top of green peppers, scoop out seeds, leaving shell intact. Blanch lids and shells in boiling water, two minutes. Plunge into cold water, drain well, set aside.

Step 2:

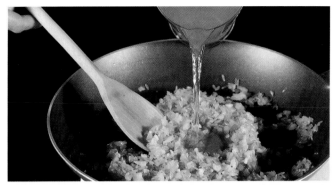

Melt margarine in a frying-pan with lid, fry onion three minutes. Stir in rice, cook until shiny, three to four minutes. Add tomato purée and stock, bring to the boil. Reduce heat, cover and simmer 15 minutes. Add mushrooms, cook a further five or six minutes, or until liquid has been absorbed. Season well, stir in nuts and soy sauce.

Step 3:

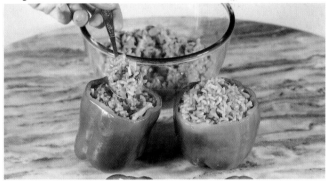

Fill peppers with rice mixture, replace lids.

To complete
Stand peppers in a roasting-pan with about 25 mm water in base. Cover with a large sheet of foil, shiny side inside , and bake at 190 °C, for 25 to 30 minutes, or until tender. Serve as a meal-in-one, with garlic bread, or as a vegetable accompaniment with chicken, meat or fish.

Serves four

Per serving: 1 147kJ; 29,7 g carbohydrate; 7,5 g protein; 13,3 g fat; 0 mg cholesterol; 5,6 g fibre
Exchanges: 2 1/2 vegetable; 1 starch; 2 fat

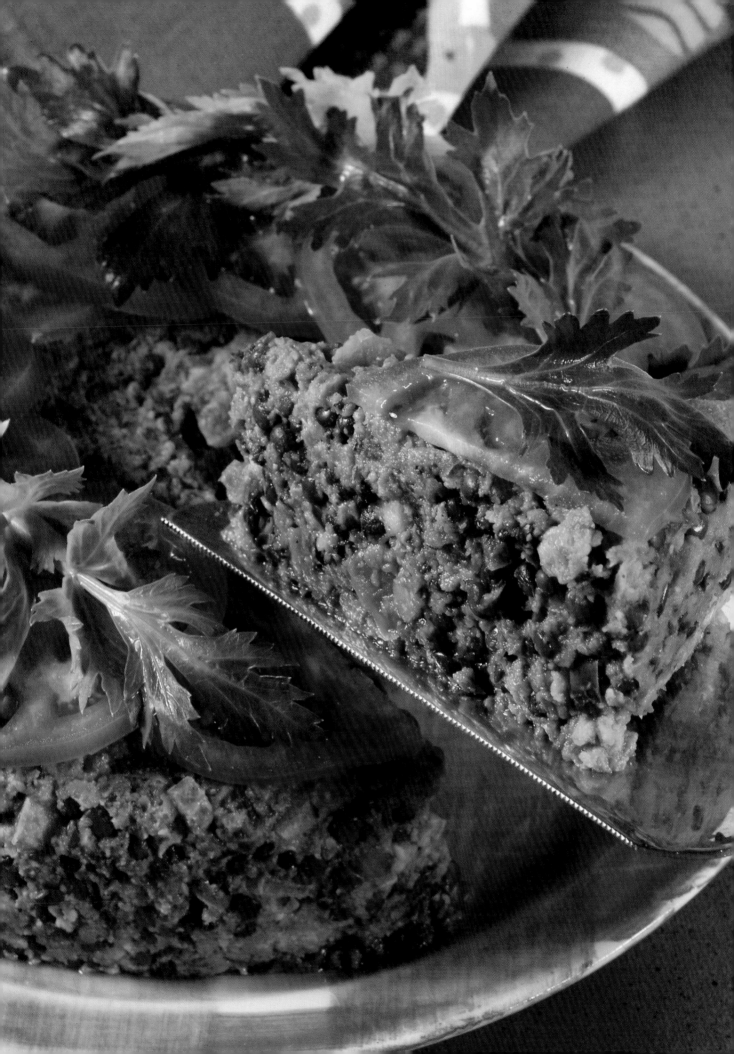

PULSES

Lentils, peas and beans are seeds from the pods of leguminous plants. For cooking purposes, the collective name Pulses refers only to the dried variety although, strictly speaking, the term embraces both fresh and dried legumes. Pulses should form a large part of the diabetic's diet — they are high in fibre, protein and minerals, but low in fat, with no cholesterol. They are economical, too, and, by soaking overnight in water to cover, the cooking time is greatly reduced. Large beans and peas require up to 12 hours' soaking; split pulses need a shorter time; small lentils (except red ones) require no soaking at all. Apart from soya beans, the protein in pulses does not contain all the essential amino acids; but, as with rice and pasta, the addition of other, incomplete protein foods will make a satisfying, flavourful meal.

LENTIL LOAF

Serve with Home-made Tomato Sauce (see Pg 90)

250 g (310 ml) brown lentils
900 ml water
12,5 ml Marmite
1 large onion, finely chopped
1 green pepper, seeded and diced
2 cloves of garlic, crushed
10 ml sunflower oil
2 tomatoes, skinned and chopped
3 celery stalks, finely chopped, including leaves
1 small apple, cored and finely diced
85 g (350 ml) wholewheat breadcrumbs
3 ml dried sage
3 ml dried origanum
10 ml finely chopped parsley
50 g (125 ml) hazel-nuts, chopped
2 eggs, beaten
salt and freshly ground black pepper to taste

Garnish
celery leaves and tomato slices

Place lentils in a saucepan, add water and Marmite, bring to the boil. Reduce heat, cover and simmer until lentils are tender and all the liquid has been absorbed, about 45 minutes. Set aside to cool. Fry onion, green pepper and garlic in heated oil until soft. Remove with slotted spoon, drain on absorbent kitchen paper towels. Add to lentils. Add tomatoes, celery, apple, bread-crumbs, herbs and nuts. Stir beaten eggs into lentil mixture, season well. Press into a lightly greased, wax-paper-base-lined 200 mm-diameter cake pan, level surface. Bake at 180 °C, about one hour, or until firm. Allow to stand 10 minutes before carefully turning out on to a heated round platter. Serve warm, cut in wedges, with vegetables or a salad.

Serves eight

Per serving: 1 125kJ; 27,4 g carbohydrate; 13,1 g protein; 9,2 g fat; 59 mg cholesterol; 9 g fibre
Exchanges: 1/2 vegetable; 1 1/2 starch; 1 fat

TUNA AND BEAN SALAD
See illustration on Pg 50

2 green apples, washed and cored
12,5 ml freshly squeezed lemon juice
185 g can tuna in brine, drained and flaked
half a small onion, grated
3 celery stalks, finely sliced
250 g sugar beans, soaked overnight, boiled until
    tender, drained

Dressing
37,5 ml olive-oil
12,5 ml vinegar
pinch of dry mustard powder
salt and freshly ground black pepper
1-2 drops liquid artificial sweetener

Garnish
watercress
4 cherry tomatoes, washed and halved

Chop apples into a bowl with lemon juice, toss well to coat, drain. Add tuna, onion, celery and beans to apple, toss gently.

Dressing
Combine all ingredients in a screw-top jar, shake well. Adjust seasoning and sweetness to taste. Pour dressing over tuna mixture, toss well. Cover, chill 30 minutes. Turn out on to a suitable serving platter or shallow salad bowl, garnish with watercress and halved cherry tomatoes. Serve with wholewheat bread.

Serves six

Per serving: 783kJ; 16,1 g carbohydrate; 11,3 g protein; 6,8 g fat; 9 mg cholesterol; 4,9 g fibre
Exchanges: 2 starch; 1 meat; 1 fat

◄ Lentil loaf

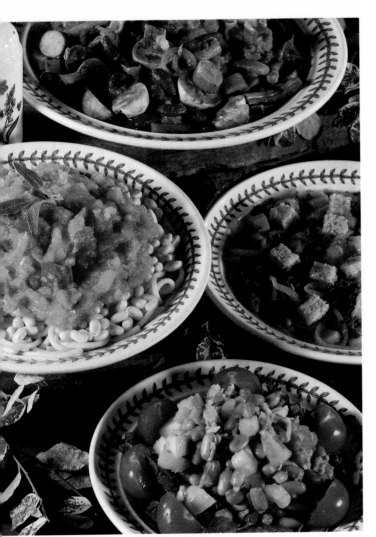

THICK LENTIL SOUP

125 g (155 ml) lentils, rinsed
5 ml salt
5 ml dried thyme
3 onions, finely sliced
3 carrots, scraped and chopped
25 ml cooking oil
60 ml finely chopped parsley
2 turnips, peeled and cubed (optional)
2 tomatoes, skinned and chopped
25 ml dry sherry (optional)

Place one litre water in a large saucepan. Add lentils, salt and thyme, bring to the boil. Reduce heat, cover and simmer 30 minutes. Drain, discard water. Add 750 ml fresh water, set aside. Sauté onions and carrots in heated oil. Reduce heat, cover and cook slowly 10 minutes, stirring occasionally. Remove with slotted spoon, drain on absorbent kitchen paper towels, add to lentils, together with remaining ingredients. Bring to the boil, reduce heat, cover and simmer a further 30 to 45 minutes, or until lentils are soft. Serve with cubes of wholewheat toast.

Serves six

Per serving: 653kJ; 16,2 g carbohydrate; 6,8 g protein; 4,3 g fat; 0 mg cholesterol; 6,7 g fibre
Exchanges: 1 vegetable; 1 starch; 1 fat

Clockwise from top: Sausage and bean stew; Thick lentil soup; Tuna and bean salad; Haricot beans with pumpkin sauce.

HARICOT BEANS WITH PUMPKIN SAUCE

250 g haricot beans, soaked overnight, drained
1 kg pumpkin, peeled, seeded and cubed
2 onions, finely chopped
1 clove of garlic, crushed
12,5 ml chopped fresh sage or 5 ml dried sage
10 ml chopped chives
10 ml tomato paste
3 tomatoes, skinned, seeded and roughly chopped
salt and freshly ground black pepper to taste

Simmer beans in water to cover, 15 minutes. Add pumpkin, onions, garlic, sage, chives and tomato paste, bring to the boil. Reduce heat, cover and simmer gently one-and-a-half hours, stirring occasionally. Add chopped tomatoes, stir until heated through. Adjust seasoning to taste. Serve hot, on a bed of pasta.

Serves four to six

Per serving: 1 483kJ; 45,4 g carbohydrate; 18,1 g protein; 2,7 g fat; 0 mg cholesterol; 25,3 g fibre
Exchanges: 1 vegetable; 4 starch

SAUSAGE AND BEAN STEW

1 onion, finely sliced
1 clove of garlic, crushed
10 ml olive-oil
375 ml home-made vegetable or chicken stock
  (see Pgs 44 and 34)
410 g can whole peeled tomatoes, undrained and
  chopped
400 g can red kidney beans, drained
250 g green beans, topped, tailed and cut into 50 mm
  lengths
3 ml dried origanum
salt and freshly ground black pepper to taste
200 g button mushrooms, wiped and halved
200 g smoked sausages, thinly sliced

Fry onion and garlic in heated oil. Pour in stock, add can of tomatoes and kidney beans, bring to the boil. Reduce heat, cover and simmer 20 minutes. Add green beans, origanum and seasoning, cover and simmer 15 minutes. Add mushrooms and sausage slices, cook five minutes more. Serve hot, on its own, or with brown rice or a baked potato.

Serves six

Per serving: 1 030kJ; 17,3 g carbohydrate; 11,2 g protein; 12,3 g fat; 17 mg cholesterol; 7,2 g fibre
Exchanges: 1 1/2 vegetable; 1/2 starch; 1 meat

PEARLED BARLEY AND LENTIL PILAFF *(Cover recipe)*

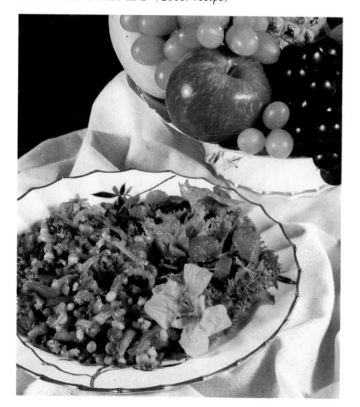

180 g (225 ml) lentils, rinsed
125 g (155 ml) pearled barley
3 ml salt
25 ml olive-oil
1 small brinjal, washed and cubed
1 red pepper *or* canned pimiento, seeded and sliced
  into strips
1 green pepper, seeded and sliced into strips
4 cloves of garlic, crushed
1 onion, sliced
250 g frozen peas
410 g can whole peeled tomatoes, drained and chopped
25 ml chopped chives
12,5 ml chopped fresh mint
25 ml chopped parsley
25 ml chopped capers
freshly ground black pepper to taste

Place lentils in a large saucepan, add one litre water, bring to the boil. Reduce heat, cover and simmer 20 to 30 minutes, until tender. Drain in colander, set aside. Boil 300 ml water in a separate saucepan, add barley and salt, boil five minutes. Drain well, add to lentils, and set aside.
Heat olive-oil in a large saucepan, fry brinjal, peppers, garlic and onion gently, about 10 minutes, stirring frequently. Add lentil mixture, peas and tomatoes, heat through gently, stirring continuously. Remove from heat, stir in remaining ingredients, toss well. Adjust seasoning to taste and serve at once, with a green salad.

Serves six

Per serving: 993kJ; 28,1 g carbohydrate; 11,7 g protein; 4,7 g fat; 0 mg cholesterol; 11 g fibre   Exchanges: 1 vegetable; 2 starch; 1 fat

MIXED BEAN *RATATOUILLE*

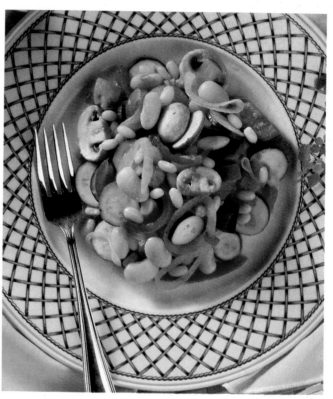

125 g small white haricot beans, soaked overnight,
  drained
125 g dried lima beans, soaked overnight, drained
10 ml olive-oil
1 large onion, sliced
2 cloves of garlic, crushed
1 red pepper *or* canned pimiento, seeded and sliced
1 green pepper, seeded and sliced into strips
500 g baby marrows, trimmed and thickly sliced
1 brinjal, washed and cut into cubes
4 large ripe tomatoes, skinned, seeded and chopped
200 g button mushrooms, wiped and halved
200 ml home-made vegetable stock (see Pg 44)
3 ml dried origanum
2 ml each freshly ground black pepper and salt

Place beans in a large saucepan, cover with water, bring to the boil, boil steadily 10 minutes, drain, discard water, rinse out saucepan. Return beans to pan, again cover with water, bring to the boil. Reduce heat, cover and simmer about one hour, or until tender. Drain and rinse, set aside. Heat olive-oil in a large, heavy-bottomed saucepan, fry onion and garlic gently, until soft. Add peppers, baby marrows, brinjals and tomatoes, cook two to three minutes, stirring frequently. Add beans, mushrooms, stock, origanum and seasoning, bring to the boil. Reduce heat, cover and simmer over low heat, 25 to 30 minutes, or until vegetables are tender but not mushy. Adjust seasoning, serve hot, with garlic rolls.

Serves six

Per serving: 782kJ; 23,6 g carbohydrate; 8,8 g protein; 3 g fat; 0 mg cholesterol; 11,1 g fibre   Exchanges: 2 vegetable; 1 1/2 starch

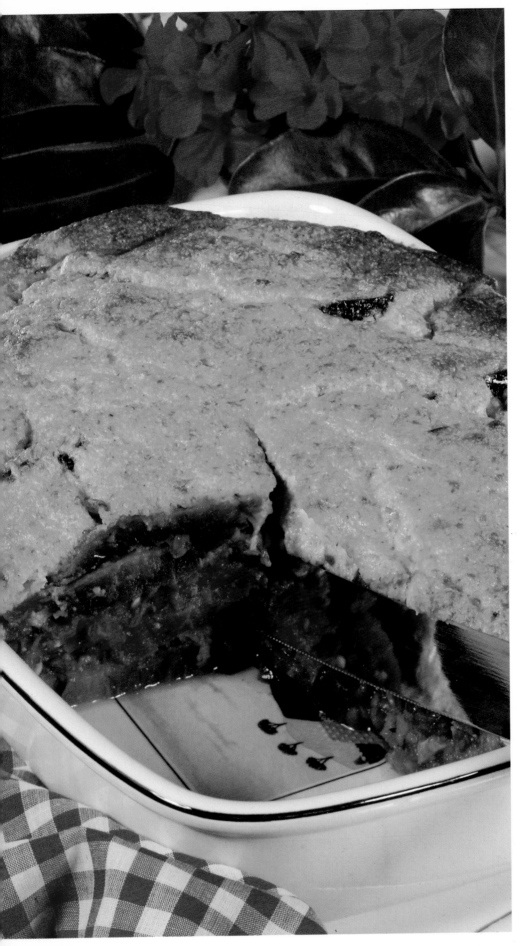

LENTIL MOUSSAKA

2 large brinjals, thickly sliced
250 g (310 ml) lentils, rinsed
1 onion, chopped
1 green pepper, seeded and
  diced
1 clove of garlic, crushed
12,5 ml olive-oil
2 canned red pimientos,
  drained and chopped
200 g button mushrooms,
  wiped and sliced
3 large ripe tomatoes, skinned
  and sliced
3 ml dried sweet basil
2 ml dried origanum
60 ml finely chopped parsley

Cheese sauce
45 g margarine
45 g (90 ml) wholewheat flour
5 ml prepared English mustard
1 ml cayenne pepper
1 ml paprika
salt and freshly ground black
  pepper
600 ml skim milk
100 g (250 ml) low-fat hard
  cheese, grated
2 eggs, separated
1 egg-white
ground nutmeg to sprinkle

Per serving: 1 236kJ; 24,2 g carbohydrate;
17,6 g protein; 10,9 g fat;
65 mg cholesterol; 10,2 g fibre
Exchanges: 1 1/2 vegetable;
1 1/2 starch; 1/2 meat; 1 1/2 fat

Step 1:

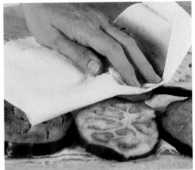

Blanch brinjal slices in boiling,
salted water, three minutes,
rinse under cold, running
water, drain on absorbent
kitchen paper towels, set aside.

Step 2:

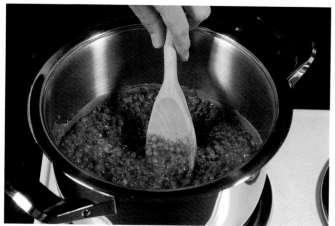

Boil lentils in lightly salted water until tender and liquid is absorbed, about 45 minutes, set aside.

Step 3:

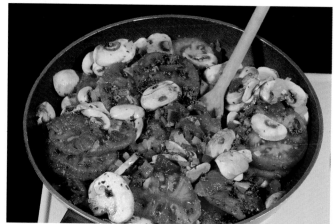

Fry onion, green pepper and garlic in heated olive-oil in a large frying-pan. Add pimientos, mushrooms, tomatoes and herbs. Cook two to three minutes, stirring gently. Remove from heat, set aside.

Step 4:

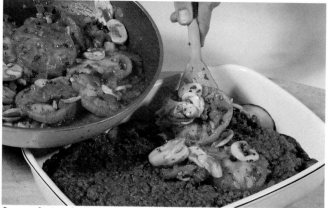

Layer brinjal slices, lentils and tomato mixture in a lightly greased 240 mm by 340 mm rectangular ovenproof dish, starting and ending with brinjal slices.

Step 5:

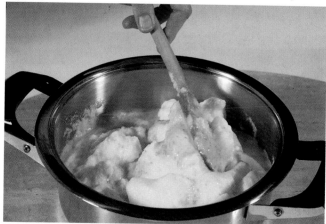

Cheese sauce: melt margarine in a saucepan, stir in flour and seasonings, cook two minutes. Remove from heat, stir in milk. Return to heat, cook, stirring continuously, until sauce boils and thickens. Cook two minutes. Remove from heat, stir in cheese. Add egg-yolks, beat well. Whip egg-whites until soft peaks form, fold into cheese sauce.

Step 6:

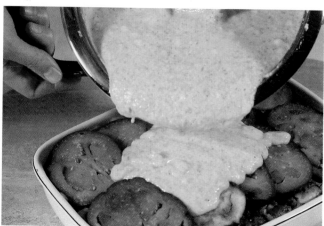

Pour cheese sauce over brinjal slices, sprinkle with nutmeg.

To complete
Bake at 190 °C, about 45 minutes, until firm and golden brown. Serve at once, with a salad and garlic bread, or wholewheat rolls.

Serves eight

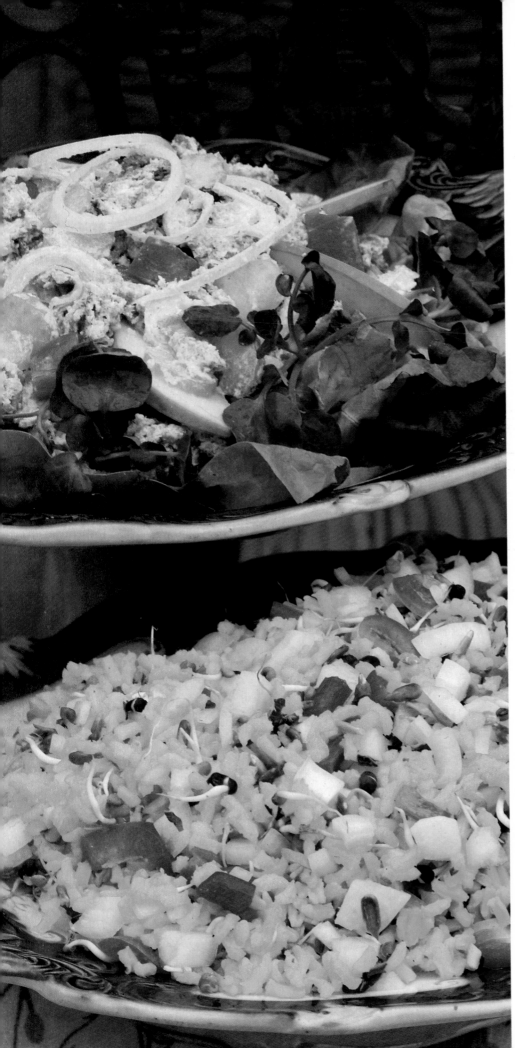

SHREDDED WHEAT SALAD

4 shredded wheat biscuits,
  broken up
250 g smooth low-fat cottage
  cheese
1 onion, sliced into rings, and
  blanched one minute
1 small green-skinned apple,
  cored and sliced into thin
  wedges
37,5 ml white wine vinegar
37,5 ml water
1 red pepper, seeded and diced
2 celery stalks, finely sliced
25 ml finely chopped parsley
salt and freshly ground black
  pepper to taste
pinch of ground nutmeg
watercress and lettuce leaves to
  serve

Blend together biscuits and
cottage cheese in a small bowl.
Add onion rings, chill 30
minutes. Combine apple
wedges with wine vinegar and
water, stir well to coat. Set
aside. Place red pepper, celery
and parsley in a bowl, add
cheese and apple mixtures, toss
well. Season with salt, pepper
and nutmeg. Turn on to a bed
of watercress and lettuce leaves,
serve at once.

Serves six

Per serving: 635kJ; 20,5 g
carbohydrate; 7,2 g protein; 4,7 g fat;
12 mg cholesterol; 1,1 g fibre
Exchanges: 1/2 vegetable; 1/2 starch;
1 meat

Back: Shredded wheat salad
Front: Sunflower rice salad

SALADS

Crisp, fresh salads are a feast for the eye and palate. Their crunchy texture oozes health and vitality, and complements any dish, be it meat, fish or poultry. Already packed with vitamins and minerals, salads can be easily transformed into a well-rounded main meal by the addition of a protein-rich food, such as cheese, eggs, fish, meat, chicken or pulses. Two things of paramount importance when preparing any salad are: fresh ingredients (ideally picked the same day), and a little imagination!

SUNFLOWER RICE SALAD

60 g (75 ml) raw brown rice
5 ml turmeric
5 ml salt
30 g (55 ml) sunflower seeds, roasted
1 onion, roughly chopped and blanched one minute
1 red pepper, seeded and diced
1 fresh chilli, seeded and finely chopped
1 clove of garlic, crushed
10 ml finely chopped parsley
freshly ground black pepper to taste
75 ml white wine vinegar
100 g bean sprouts

Cook rice in boiling water with turmeric and salt until tender, about 20 minutes, drain well, allow to cool. Combine with seeds, onion, red pepper, chilli, garlic and parsley, season with more salt if necessary, and black pepper. Pour wine vinegar over salad, toss well. Cover and refrigerate until well chilled. Stir in bean sprouts just before serving.

Serves four

Per serving: 485kJ; 13,9 g carbohydrate; 4,6 g protein; 4,6 g fat; 0 mg cholesterol; 2,5 g fibre
Exchanges: 1 vegetable; 1/2 starch; 1 fat

CURRIED APPLE COLESLAW

175 ml low-fat plain yoghurt
25 ml home-made chutney (see Pg 99)
1-2 drops liquid artificial sweetener
3 ml medium curry-powder
1 ml ground ginger
3 ml lemon juice
half a cabbage, finely shredded
1 large Granny Smith apple, washed and grated
salt and freshly ground pepper to taste

Whisk together first six ingredients. Combine cabbage and apple in a glass salad bowl, pour over yoghurt mixture, toss well. Season well. Cover and chill 30 minutes before serving.

Serves six

Per serving: 201kJ; 7,9 g carbohydrate; 2 g protein; 0,7 g fat; 2 mg cholesterol; 1,5 g fibre
Exchanges: 1 1/2 vegetable

CHICKEN AND BREAD-CUBE SALAD

500 g chicken breast fillets
375 ml water
3 ml chicken stock powder
1 onion, finely chopped
25 ml freshly squeezed lemon juice
10 ml olive-oil
5 ml dried sweet basil
3 ml dried origanum
1 ml salt
1 clove of garlic, crushed
4 slices day-old rye bread, toasted and cubed
2 tomatoes, roughly chopped
3 celery stalks, finely sliced

Poach chicken fillets in water with stock powder and onion until tender, 10 to 15 minutes. Remove chicken with a slotted spoon, reserve cooking liquid. Allow chicken to cool, cut into bite-sized pieces, set aside. Combine next seven ingredients in a mixing-bowl, stir well. Add chicken, tomatoes, celery and 60 ml reserved cooking liquid, toss well. Cover and chill one hour before serving. Serve with lettuce leaves and a baked potato as a main meal.

Serves four

Per serving: 1 109kJ; 18,7 g carbohydrate; 29,3 g protein; 7,4 g fat; 68 mg cholesterol; 3,7 g fibre
Exchanges: 1 vegetable; 1 starch; 3 meat; 1/2 fat

APPLE AND SPROUT SALAD

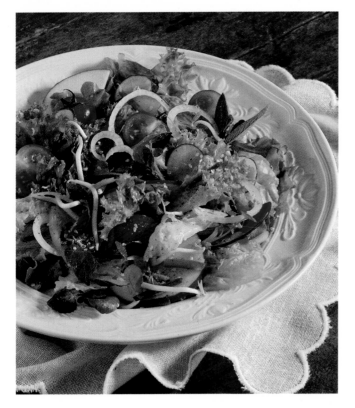

To remove the harsh taste of a raw onion, blanch in boiling water for one minute, drain and plunge into cold water immediately. Drain well. The same may be done with raw red and green peppers if you find them difficult to digest.

one-third English cucumber, washed and thinly sliced
4 spring onions, diagonally sliced
half a red pepper, seeded and cut julienne
6-8 cherry tomatoes, washed and halved
half a red-skinned apple, cored and sliced into rings
half a green-skinned apple, cored and sliced into rings
120 g packet California salad mix (salad greens)
half an onion, finely sliced into rings, and blanched one minute
50 g bean sprouts
2 radishes, washed and finely sliced
10 ml sesame seeds
10 ml digestive bran

To complete
freshly squeezed lemon juice
freshly ground black pepper

Combine all salad ingredients in a large bowl, toss gently. Turn into a serving dish or plate, sprinkle with sesame seeds and bran. Drizzle lemon juice over salad, toss well, add pepper to taste. Serve at once.

Serves four to six

Per serving: 271kJ; 9,8 g carbohydrate; 2,4 g protein; 1,5 g fat; 0 mg cholesterol; 3,1 g fibre
Exchanges: 1 vegetable

56

RED KIDNEY BEAN SLAW

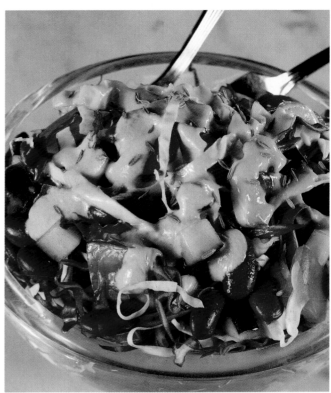

If red and yellow peppers are not available, use green only.

500 ml finely shredded green cabbage (3-4 leaves)
500 ml finely shredded red cabbage (3-4 leaves)
190 ml finely diced cucumber with skin
half a green pepper, seeded and cut into large squares
half a yellow pepper, seeded and cut into large squares
1 red pepper, seeded and cut into large squares
425 g can red kidney beans, drained

Yoghurt dressing
60 ml low-fat plain yoghurt
25 ml tomato cocktail *or* tomato purée
few drops liquid artificial sweetener
12,5 ml lemon juice
3 ml cumin seeds
salt and freshly ground black pepper to taste

Place all ingredients in a bowl. Combine dressing ingredients, adjust seasoning to taste. Pour dressing over salad, toss well. Cover and chill thoroughly before serving.

Serves eight

Per serving: 363kJ; 11,2 g carbohydrate; 5,4 g protein; 0,4 g fat; 0 mg cholesterol; 5,2 g fibre
Exchanges: 1/2 vegetable; 1/2 starch

LETTUCE, OLIVE AND ORANGE SALAD

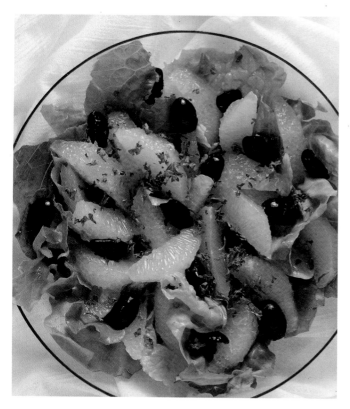

5 large oranges, thickly peeled and segmented,
   juice reserved
8 black olives, halved and pitted
37,5 ml reserved orange juice
25 ml white wine vinegar
5 ml paprika
2 ml freshly ground black pepper
1 clove of garlic, crushed
1 small lettuce, washed
12,5 ml finely chopped parsley

Place orange segments and olives in a glass bowl. Add next five ingredients, stir gently. Cover and refrigerate, one hour. Drain , discard liquid. Line a shallow glass salad bowl with lettuce leaves. Top with orange segments and olives. Sprinkle with parsley, serve at once, as a starter, or with chicken or pork.

Serves six

Per serving: 494kJ; 21,7 g carbohydrate; 2,4 g protein; 1 g fat; 0 mg cholesterol; 5,9 g fibre
Exchanges: 1 fruit

NEW POTATO SALAD

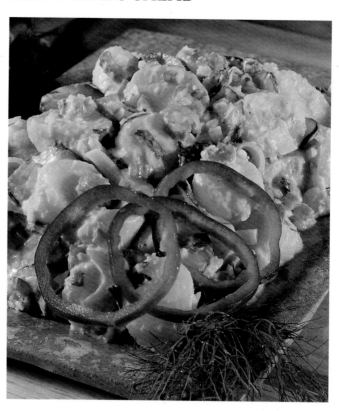

A good accompaniment to grilled or braaied meat, fish or poultry. Diabetic Mayonnaise may be substituted for the yoghurt dressing, if preferred (see Pg 93).

500 g new potatoes, scrubbed
1 green pepper, washed
2 celery stalks, sliced, including leaves
1 small head of fennel, sliced and leaves reserved
   (optional)
1 onion, finely chopped and blanched one minute
one-quarter English cucumber, finely sliced
150 ml low-fat plain yoghurt
5 ml finely grated lemon rind
5 ml prepared French mustard
pinch of cayenne pepper
salt and freshly ground black pepper to taste

Cook potatoes in boiling salted water until just tender, but still firm, about 15 minutes. Rinse under cold, running water, pat dry. Remove skins, cut potatoes in half, leave to cool. Slice off two rings of green pepper, reserve. Seed and dice remainder. Combine all vegetables in a bowl, toss gently. Combine remaining ingredients, beat well with a spoon. Pour dressing over salad, toss to coat. Pile on to serving plate, garnish with green pepper rings and reserved fennel leaves, serve at once.

Serves six

Per serving: 440kJ; 20,2 g carbohydrate; 3,4 g protein; 0,6 g fat; 2 mg cholesterol; 2,1 g fibre
Exchanges: 1 starch

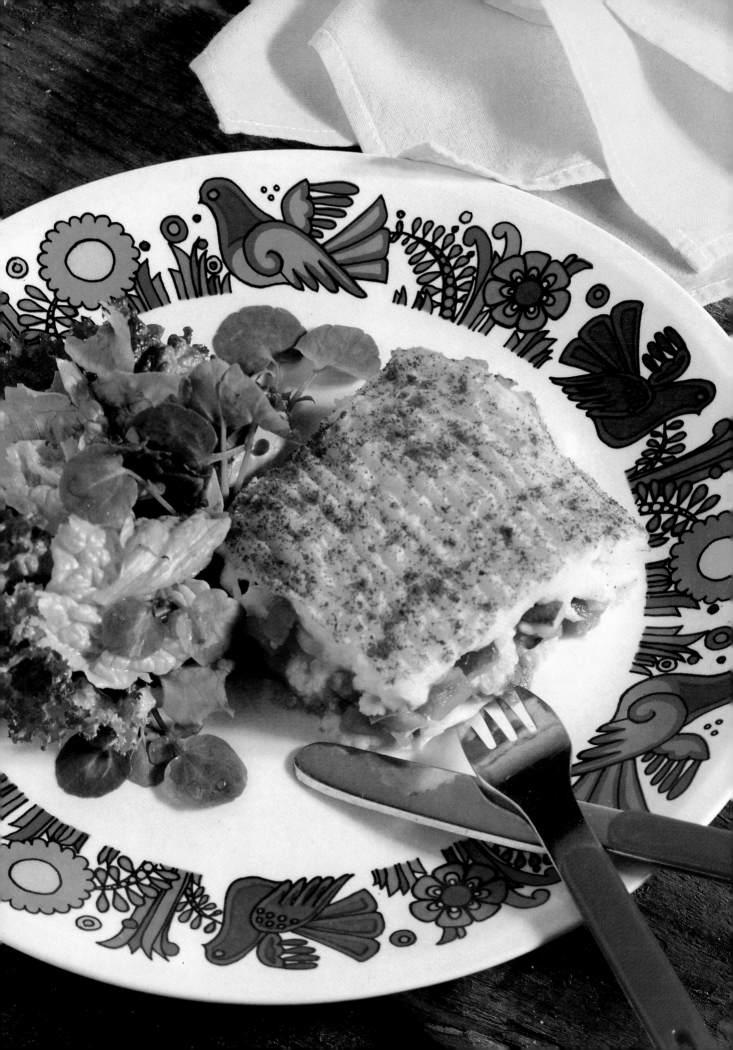

LUNCH AND SUPPER DISHES

These simple-to-prepare dishes are mainly vegetarian meals-in-one, requiring at most a salad or crusty wholewheat roll as accompaniment. Try the open sandwiches or tasty pasties for the school lunchbox, office snack or weekend picnic.

SALAD AND POTATO PIE

1 kg large potatoes, scrubbed
12,5 ml wholewheat flour
50 ml skim milk
1 egg, beaten
60 ml low-fat plain yoghurt
25 ml finely chopped red herbs (optional)
4 ml salt
2 ml ground nutmeg
100 g cabbage, finely shredded
100 g baby fresh *or* canned sweetcorn, sliced
200 g English cucumber, washed and cut into 25 mm-long sticks
3 tomatoes, skinned, seeded and chopped
half a green pepper, seeded and diced
half a red pepper, seeded and diced
freshly ground black pepper to taste
3 ml paprika

Prick potatoes well, bake at 200 °C, one hour, or in microwave oven on 100% (High) power, four minutes for each potato, until tender. Allow to cool slightly, remove skin and mash potatoes. Set aside. Beat together flour, milk, egg, yoghurt, red herbs, 2 ml salt and nutmeg. Add mashed potatoes, mix well.
Spray inside of a deep, 260 mm by 180 mm ovenproof dish with non-stick spray. Line base and sides with half potato mixture. Fill dish with cabbage, corn, cucumber, tomatoes and peppers, season with remaining salt and black pepper. Carefully spread remaining potato mixture over vegetables, covering them completely. Mark surface with a fork and sprinkle with paprika. Bake at 200 °C, about 20 minutes, until lightly browned and firm. Serve cut into squares, with a green salad.

Serves six

Per serving: 897kJ; 39,6 g carbohydrate; 6,8 g protein; 1,7 g fat; 39 mg cholesterol; 5,4 g fibre
Exchanges: 1 vegetable; 2 starch

PIZZA TOMATO SAUCE

Sufficient for four pizzas. Make the full quantity, refrigerate for up to one week, or freeze for up to one month. May be used as a sauce for burgers, a base for Bolognese Sauce, or a topping for baked fish or baked potatoes.

12,5 ml olive-oil
3 large onions, finely chopped
5 cloves of garlic, crushed
2 x 410 g cans whole peeled tomatoes, liquid reserved, chopped
150 ml dry white wine *or* water
105 g can *or* 2 x 65 g cans tomato paste
25 ml white wine vinegar
3 ml cayenne pepper
5 ml paprika
10 ml dried sweet basil
4 ml liquid artificial sweetener *or* to taste
salt and freshly ground black pepper

Heat olive-oil in a large, heavy-bottomed saucepan, fry onions and garlic, four to five minutes. Add remaining ingredients, bring to the boil. Reduce heat, simmer uncovered, about 30 minutes, stirring frequently, until thick and well reduced. Allow to cool.

Makes 4 x 250 ml

Per 250 ml: 653kJ; 18,2 g carbohydrate; 4 g protein; 4 g fat; 0 mg cholesterol; 4,9 g fibre
Exchanges: 3 vegetable

◄ Salad and potato pie

OPEN SANDWICHES

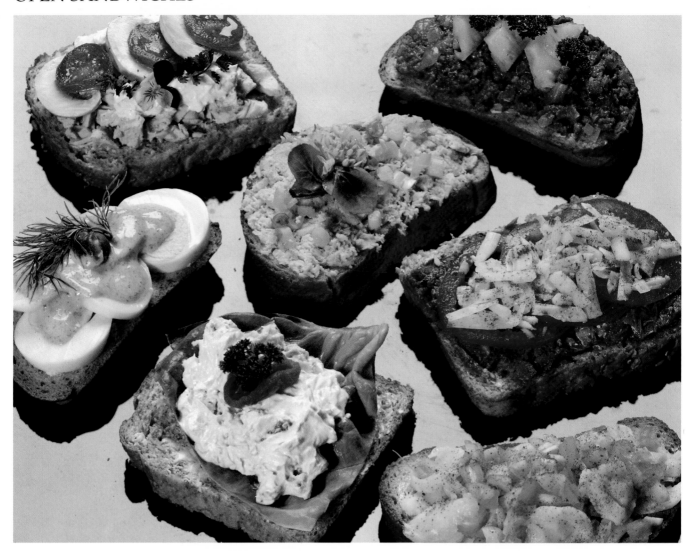

Fillings may also be used for closed sandwiches for
lunchboxes, office snack-packs or travel-fare. Sandwiches
which contain cooked meat, fish or cheese freeze well. Those
containing fresh fruit, salad greens, mayonnaise, cottage
cheese, hard-boiled eggs and tomatoes should not be frozen,
but may be refrigerated overnight, if necessary.

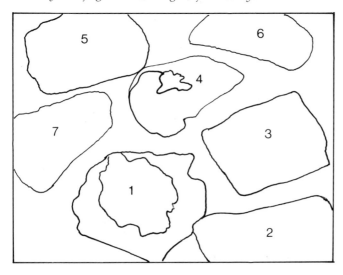

rye bread *or* wholewheat bread, sliced
low-fat spread

Suggested fillings

1. lettuce leaf; smooth low-fat cottage cheese; chopped
   dried apricots

2. flaked cooked hake; chopped celery; paprika

3. drained mashed pilchards; tomato slices; grated low-
   fat cheese; paprika

4. drained flaked salmon; chopped spring onions

5. chopped cooked chicken; tomato slices; sliced
   button mushrooms; smooth low-fat cottage cheese

6. cooked savoury mince; chopped fresh pineapple;
   parsley

7. sliced hard-boiled egg; yoghurt and curry-
   powder; capers; watercress or fresh herbs

Spread bread slices with low-fat spread. Top with any of
the suggested fillings, season to taste and garnish as
desired. Serve at once.

(Values dependant on filling chosen)

MEXICAN CHILLI BEAN PIZZA

425 g can chilli beans, drained
1 small onion, finely chopped
5 ml cumin seeds
2 ml chilli-powder *or* to taste
1 ml salt
1 clove of garlic, crushed
1 prepared Wholewheat Pizza Crust (see Pg 66)
2 large tomatoes, finely chopped
1 bunch spring onions, finely chopped
1 green pepper, seeded and diced
100 g (250 ml) low-fat hard cheese, grated
4 g (10 ml) grated Parmesan cheese
freshly ground black pepper to taste

Combine beans, onion, cumin, chilli-powder, salt and
garlic in a bowl, spread over prepared crust, leaving a
12 mm border. Sprinkle tomatoes, spring onions and
green pepper over bean mixture, top with cheeses and
pepper. Bake at 240 °C, about 15 minutes. Serve hot.
Serves six

Per serving: 1 072kJ; 32,3 g carbohydrate; 15 g protein; 5,2 g fat;
8 mg cholesterol; 8,4 g fibre
Exchanges: 1/2 vegetable; 2 starch; 1/2 meat

VEGETABLE PIZZA

250 g broccoli florets
150 g carrots, scraped and cut julienne
100 g snow peas
100 g baby marrows, trimmed and cut julienne

White sauce
12 g (25 ml) cornflour
300 ml skim milk
10 g (25 ml) grated Parmesan cheese
2 ml salt
freshly ground black pepper to taste

To complete
4 spring onions, finely sliced
15 ml chopped fresh basil *or* 5 ml dried sweet basil
one-quarter quantity Pizza Tomato Sauce (see Pg 59)
1 prepared Wholewheat Pizza Crust (see Pg 66)
25 g (60 ml) Mozzarella *or* low-fat hard cheese, grated

Blanch broccoli, carrots, peas and baby marrow in
boiling water, five minutes. Drain, rinse under cold,
running water. Pat dry, set aside.

White sauce
Cook cornflour and milk in a saucepan over medium
heat, stirring all the time, until mixture boils and
thickens. Stir in remaining ingredients, remove heat.
Add blanched vegetables, spring onions, basil, stir well.
Spread Pizza Tomato Sauce over prepared Wholewheat
Pizza Crust. Spoon vegetable mixture over sauce.
Sprinkle with cheese. Bake at 240 °C, 12 minutes. Allow
to stand five minutes before cutting.

Serves six

Per serving: 1 133kJ; 38,6 g carbohydrate; 14,2 g protein; 3,8 g fat;
6 mg cholesterol; 9,2 g fibe Exchanges: 1 1/2 vegetable; 1 1/2 starch

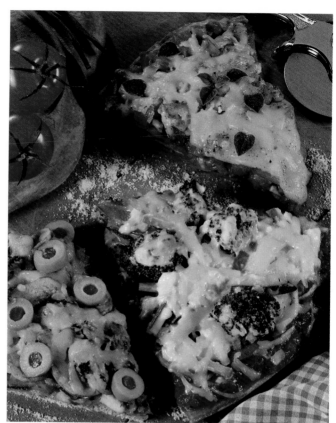

Clockwise from top: Mexican chilli bean pizza; Vegetable pizza;
Chicken and mushroom pizza

CHICKEN AND MUSHROOM PIZZA

250 g skinned, boned chicken breast, diced
200 g button mushrooms, wiped and sliced
1 onion, finely chopped
3 cloves of garlic, crushed
37,5 ml finely chopped parsley
25 mm-piece fresh ginger, peeled and grated
10 ml soy sauce
60 ml skim milk
salt and freshly ground black pepper to taste
50 g (125 ml) low-fat hard cheese, grated
1 prepared Wholewheat Pizza Crust (see Pg 66)
4 g (10 ml) grated Parmesan cheese
5 stuffed green olives, halved, for garnish

Spray a large frying-pan with non-stick spray, heat well.
Fry chicken to brown lightly. Add mushrooms, onion,
garlic and parsley, sauté lightly, three to four minutes
over medium heat. Add ginger, soy sauce and milk,
bring to the boil, cook, uncovered, until liquid has
reduced. Adjust seasoning to taste. Sprinkle half grated
cheese over Wholewheat Pizza Crust. Top with chicken
mixture. Sprinkle remaining grated cheese and
Parmesan cheese over chicken, garnish with halved,
stuffed olives. Bake at 240 °C, 12 minutes. Allow to
stand five minutes before cutting.

Serves six

Per serving: 897kJ; 24,4 g carbohydrate; 16,8 g protein; 4,3 g fat;
26 mg cholesterol; 3,9 g fibre
Exchanges: 1/2 vegetable; 1 1/2 starch; 1 1/2 meat

CORNISH PASTIES

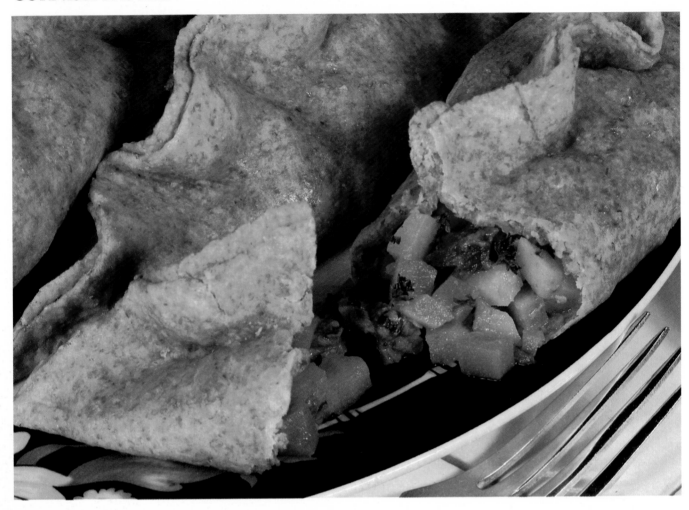

The wholewheat shortcrust pastry has a lovely, light texture, and, if preferred, may be used instead of the flaky pastry suggested for the Christmas mince pies. Also use it for the Sweet Fruit Tartlets on Pg 83 and Apple Triangles on Pg 72.

Wholewheat pastry
**250 g (500 ml) wholewheat flour, sifted and husks
    replaced**
125 g (250 ml) flour, sifted
125 g margarine
about 250 ml iced water to mix

Filling
**250 g rump steak, trimmed, thinly sliced and cut into
    small cubes**
1 medium turnip, peeled and finely diced
1 medium carrot, scraped and finely diced
1 medium potato, peeled and finely diced
37,5 ml finely chopped parsley
salt and freshly ground black pepper to taste

To complete
1 egg-white, lightly beaten
25 ml skim milk

Wholewheat pastry
Combine flours in a large mixing-bowl. Rub in

margarine until mixture resembles fine breadcrumbs. Alternatively, process in food processor. Gradually add enough iced water to make a firm, pliable dough, which sticks together and leaves the sides of the bowl clean. Turn out on to a lightly floured surface, knead until smooth. Wrap in clingwrap, chill 30 minutes in the refrigerator.

Filling
Combine meat, vegetables, parsley and seasoning in a bowl, set aside. Roll out pastry thinly on a floured surface, cut into 12 rounds of 120 mm-diameter each. Spoon 50 ml to 60 ml filling into centre of each round, wet edges with a mixture of egg-white and milk, fold pastry in half over filling. Stand with join uppermost, flute along join. Stand on lightly greased baking tray, brush with egg-white and milk mixture, prick with a fork. Bake at 180 °C, 25 to 30 minutes. Serve hot or cold, with Worcestershire sauce, a thin gravy or Home-made Tomato Sauce (see Pg 92), or wrap securely and freeze for up to three months.

Makes 12

Per pasty: 965kJ; 23,7 g carbohydrate; 9,3 g protein; 9,7 g fat; 13 mg
cholesterol; 3,8 g fibre
Exchanges: 1 1/2 starch; 1/2 meat; 2 fat

CABBAGE ROLL-UPS

8 large green cabbage leaves,
  hard stalks removed
100 g speckled sugar beans,
  soaked overnight, drained
410 g can whole peeled
  tomatoes, undrained
3 cloves of garlic, crushed
60 ml white wine vinegar
25 drops liquid artificial
  sweetener
150 g baby marrows, trimmed
  and diced
15 ml olive-oil
salt and freshly ground black
  pepper to taste
25 ml finely chopped fresh
  herbs
6 g (15 ml) grated Parmesan
  cheese
125 ml water

Simmer cabbage leaves in a
large saucepan of boiling water,
eight to 10 minutes, or until
limp, drain well, set aside. Boil
beans in water to cover, about
45 minutes, or until tender,
drain well. Place next four
ingredients in an electric
blender or a food processor,
blend until smooth. Sauté baby
marrows in heated olive-oil,
five minutes. Add half tomato
mixture and seasoning. Simmer,
uncovered, about 10 minutes,
until well reduced. Stir in herbs,
cheese and beans.
Divide baby marrow mixture
between the eight cabbage
leaves. Fold two sides over
filling, roll up cabbage leaf into
a parcel. Arrange roll-ups in a
lightly greased ovenproof dish,
pour over water and remaining
tomato mixture. Cover and
bake at 180 °C, 30 to 40 minutes.
Serve at once, with brown rice
or mashed potato.

Serves four or eight

Per roll-up: 521kJ; 11,5 g carbohydrate;
4,9 g protein; 5,1 g fat; 2 mg
cholesterol; 5,4 g fibre
Exchanges: 1 vegetable; 1 starch; 1 fat

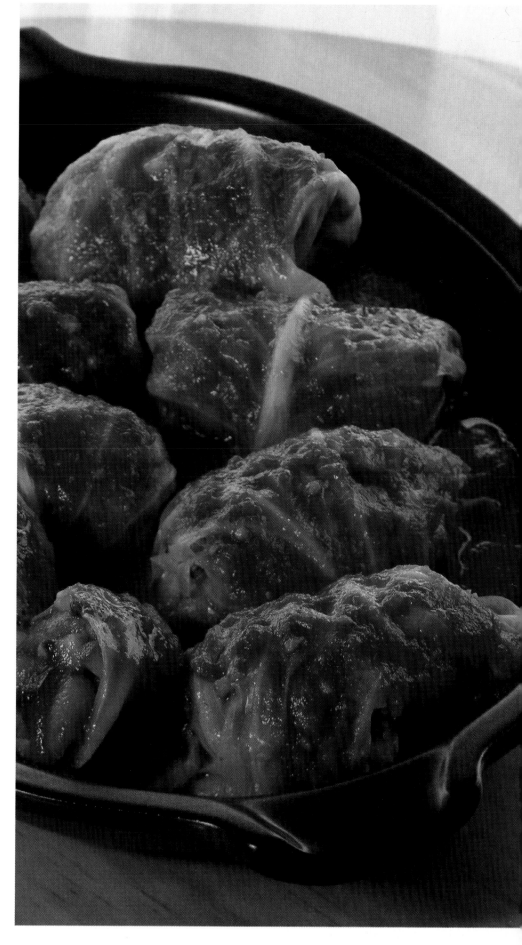

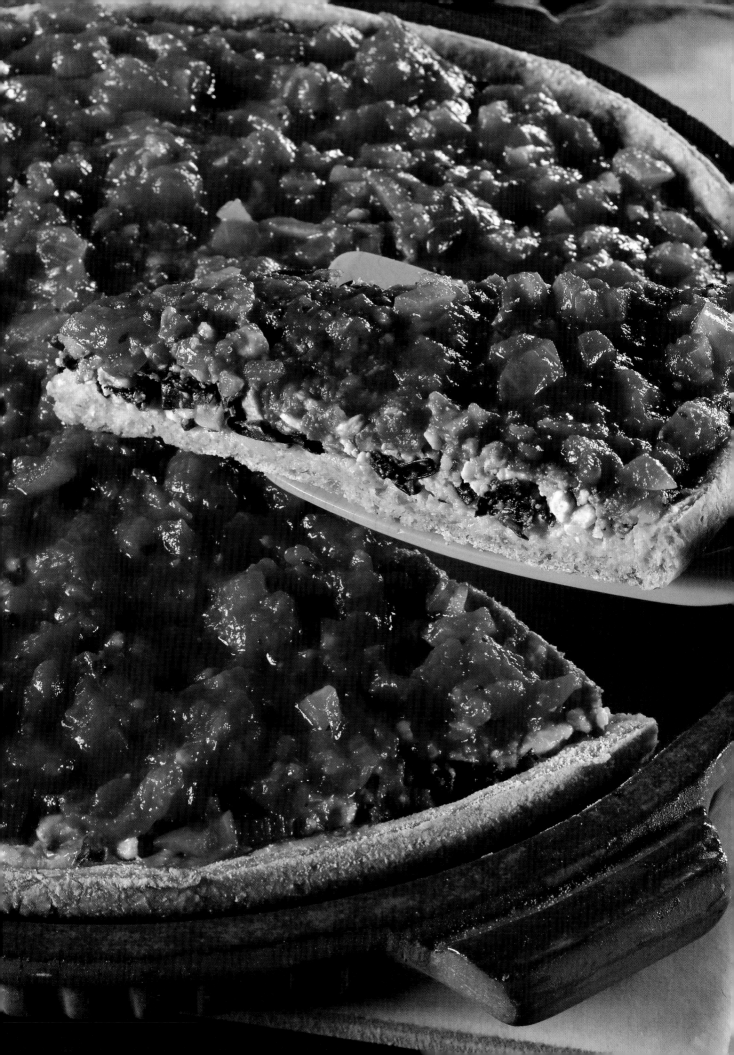

SPINACH AND RICOTTA PIZZA

1 small onion, finely chopped
125 g fresh spinach, finely shredded
250 g Ricotta cheese *or* 2 x 250 g tubs chunky low-fat
   cottage cheese
50 g (125 ml) low-fat hard cheese, grated
salt and freshly ground black pepper to taste
1 egg-white, lightly beaten
1 prepared Wholewheat Pizza Crust (see Pg 66)
one-quarter quantity Pizza Tomato Sauce (see Pg 59)
5 ml grated Parmesan cheese

Per serving: 972kJ; 27,1 g carbohydrate; 13,3 g protein; 6,3 g fat;
16 mg cholesterol; 4,5 g fibre
Exchanges: 1 vegetable; 1 1/2 starch; 2 meat

Step 1:

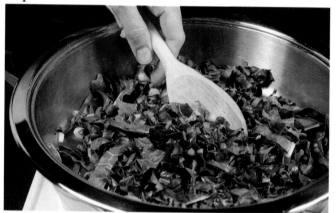

Spray a large frying-pan with non-stick spray, fry onion
three minutes over medium heat. Add spinach, sauté
one minute.

Step 2:

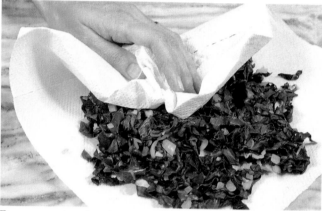

Remove spinach mixture to absorbent kitchen paper
towels, squeeze until dry.

Step 3:

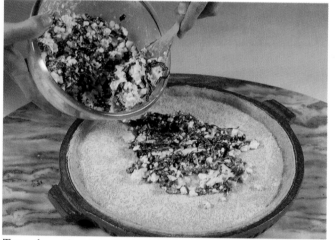

Transfer spinach mixture to a bowl, combine with
cheeses, seasoning and egg-white. Spread over
Wholewheat Pizza Crust.

Step 4:

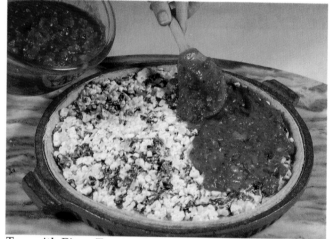

Top with Pizza Tomato Sauce, spreading right to edges.

To complete
Sprinkle with Parmesan cheese, bake at 240 °C, 15 to
20 minutes. Allow to stand five minutes before cutting.

Serves six

SPANISH OMELETTE

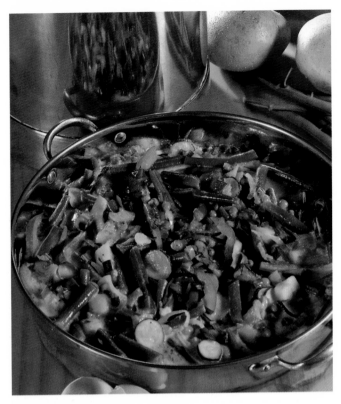

25 ml olive-oil
1 large onion, finely chopped
2 cloves of garlic, crushed
100 g baby marrows, trimmed and sliced
half a green pepper, seeded and sliced julienne
250 ml frozen green peas, thawed
2 eggs
2 egg-whites
3 ml salt
freshly ground black pepper
1 cooked potato, skinned and diced
125 g green beans, sliced, blanched five minutes,
  drained
2 tomatoes, skinned and chopped
10 ml chopped fresh herbs
3 ml dried thyme
10 ml margarine

Heat olive-oil in a large frying-pan, fry onion and garlic
until soft. Add baby marrows and green pepper, fry
gently 10 minutes.
Stir in peas. Remove with slotted spoon, drain on
absorbent kitchen paper towels, set aside. Whisk
together eggs, egg-whites and seasoning in a mixing-
bowl. Add fried mixture together with remaining
ingredients, except margarine.
Add margarine to any oil remaining in frying-pan, heat
until melted. Pour in egg mixture, cook three to four
minutes until beginning to set, stirring occasionally.
Cover and cook gently until firm, or place under
preheated griller to brown top. Serve at once, cut into
large wedges.

Serves four

WHOLEWHEAT PIZZA CRUST

*This recipe is enough for four pizzas. If you make one only,
freeze remaining dough for up to three months. To thaw,
refrigerate overnight, bring to room temperature, and roll out.
Alternatively, make all four pizza bases and freeze, layered,
with greaseproof paper between. Pizzas may also be prepared
complete with fillings, and frozen, unbaked, for up to one
month. Bake straight from freezer, allowing extra time.*

20 g (30 ml) active dry yeast *or* 2 cakes fresh yeast
650 ml lukewarm water
475 g (950 ml) wholewheat flour, sifted and husks
  replaced
250 g (500 ml) flour, sifted
3 ml salt
25 drops liquid artificial sweetener
10 ml olive-oil
25 ml yellow mealie-meal

Combine yeast and water, set aside about 15 minutes in
a warm, draught-free place. Sift together 375 g (750 ml)
wholewheat flour, flour and salt into a large mixing-
bowl. Make a well in centre, add sweetener, olive-oil
and yeast mixture, mix well to form a dough. Add
remaining wholewheat flour gradually, kneading well.
Turn out dough on to a lightly floured surface, knead
well. Return to lightly oiled bowl. Oil top of dough
lightly, cover bowl and leave in warm, draught-free
place until doubled in bulk, about one hour.
Punch down dough, divide into four equal parts. Roll
out each into a 300 mm circle, place on lightly greased
baking trays. Crimp edges to form a small border.
Sprinkle lightly with mealie-meal. Cover, leave to rise
until doubled in bulk, about 30 minutes. Top with
desired topping, bake at 240 °C, on lowest shelf of oven
(to gain maximum heat from underneath), 12 to
15 minutes.

Makes four pizza bases

Per pizza base: 2 884kJ; 123,9 g carbohydrate; 23,8 g protein;
6,2 g fat; 0 mg cholesterol; 18 g fibre
Exchanges: 9 starch

◄ Per serving: 967kJ; 18,5 g carbohydrate; 9,1 g protein; 11,9 g fat;
117 mg cholesterol; 5,4 g fibre
Exchanges: 2 vegetable; 1/2 meat; 2 fat

LEEK AND RICOTTA MONEY-BAGS

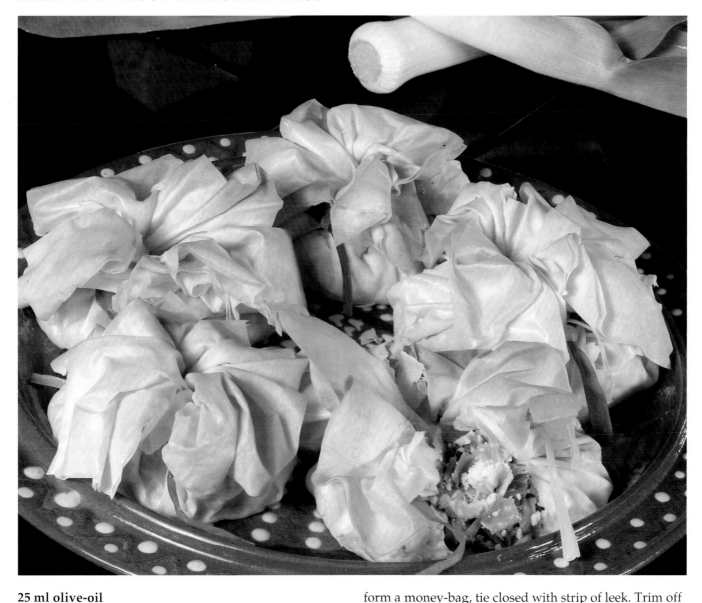

25 ml olive-oil
60 g margarine, melted
4 leeks, trimmed, halved lengthwise and washed
1 large onion, finely chopped
2 cloves of garlic, crushed
3 ml pinch of herbs
2 ml salt
freshly ground black pepper to taste
pinch grated nutmeg
200 g Ricotta cheese, crumbled
12 sheets phyllo pastry, each 270 mm-square, thawed
strips of leek *or* spring onion leaves for tying

Heat olive-oil and half margarine in a heavy-bottomed frying-pan. Cut leeks into 10 mm lengths, add to pan with onion, garlic, herbs, salt, pepper and nutmeg, fry gently 10 minutes, stirring all the time. Stir in cheese, continue cooking two more minutes. Transfer mixture to a bowl, allow to cool. Place two sheets of phyllo pastry on top of each other, on a clean, dry, work surface. Divide leek mixture into six equal parts, place one part in centre of pastry square. Bring up corners to centre to form a money-bag, tie closed with strip of leek. Trim off excess pastry with scissors. Repeat with remaining phyllo and leek mixture, making six bags in all. Arrange money-bags on a baking-tray, brush with remaining melted margarine, bake at 190 °C, for 25 to 30 minutes, until pastry is crisp and golden brown. Serve at once, with a tomato and lettuce salad.

Serves six

Per serving: 3 338kJ; 71,1 g carbohydrate; 11,7 g protein; 50,5 g fat; 10 mg cholesterol; 3,6 g fibre
Exchanges: 2 starch; 1 meat; 5 fat

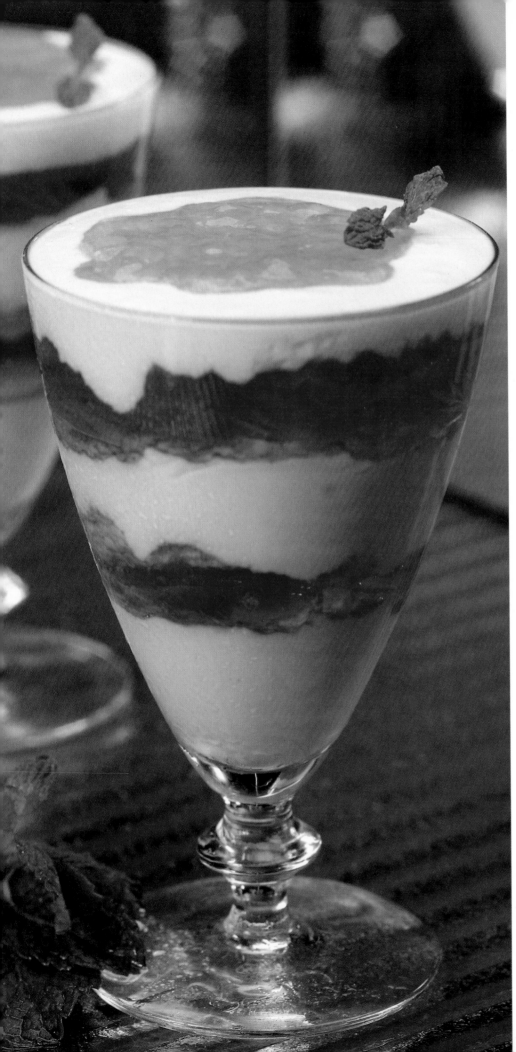

STRIPED GREEN GLORY

Use different-flavoured cordials to vary the colour of the stripes, or substitute diabetic jelly for the cordial and gelatine mixture.

10 g (15 ml) gelatine
475 ml water
37,5 ml diabetic lime cordial
12,5 ml freshly squeezed lemon juice
few drops of green food colouring
4 ml liquid artificial sweetener *or* to taste
250 ml low-fat plain yoghurt
250 g tub low-fat smooth cottage cheese
mint sprigs to decorate

Soak gelatine in 37,5 ml water, dissolve over a saucepan of simmering water, or in the microwave oven. Add remaining water, stir well. Leave to cool. Stir in cordial, lemon juice, colouring and 1 ml sweetener. Chill in refrigerator until beginning to thicken. Combine yoghurt and cottage cheese, beat well.
Add 3 ml sweetener. Spoon cheese mixture alternately with thickened jelly mixture into three tall serving glasses, chill in refrigerator until ready to serve. Decorate with mint sprigs.

Serves three

Per serving: 626kJ; 8,3 g carbohydrate; 17,3 g protein; 5 g fat; 17 mg cholesterol; 0 g fibre
Exchanges: 2 meat

DESSERTS

To appease the cravings of the most demanding sweet tooth, these mouth-watering desserts have been designed for maximum eye and palate appeal, with greatly reduced fat and kilojoule content. Liquid artificial sweetener is used in all the recipes. It's heat-stable, doesn't lose its sweetness when cooked or baked, and is kilojoule-free – an added bonus. Don't over-indulge – satisfy your hunger with the main meal, leaving just enough space for a tantalising after-dinner treat. Remember to serve small portions and include the nutritional content in your daily dietetic calculations.

NO-BAKE MILK TART

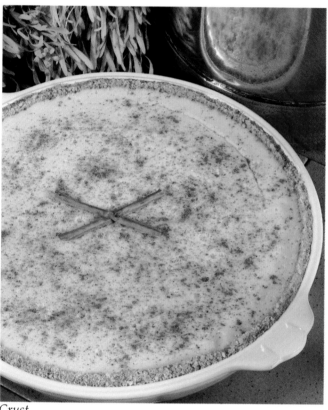

Crust
200 g packet cream cracker biscuits, crushed
110 g margarine, melted
2 ml liquid artificial sweetener *or* to taste
2 ml ground mixed spice

Filling
700 ml skim milk
1 stick cinnamon
37 g (75 ml) cornflour
3 eggs
2 ml liquid artificial sweetener *or* to taste
5 ml vanilla essence
2 ml almond essence
ground nutmeg *or* cinnamon to sprinkle

Crust
Combine ingredients, press into a lightly greased 230 mm-diameter pie-plate. Chill in refrigerator.

Filling
Measure off 75 ml milk, set aside. Heat remaining milk with cinnamon to just below boiling point. Remove from heat. Stir cornflour into reserved milk until smooth, add strained hot milk. Return to heat, bring to the boil, stirring continuously. Cook, stirring, about five minutes, until thick and smooth. Remove from heat, beat in eggs, sweetener and essences. Whisk over a saucepan of gently simmering water, three to four minutes – don't cook too quickly or the eggs will curdle. Strain through a fine sieve into prepared crust, sprinkle with ground nutmeg. Allow to cool. Refrigerate until set, at least three to four hours, or until ready to serve.

Serves 12

Per serving: 863kJ; 19,4 g carbohydrate; 5,6 g protein; 12,2 g fat; 70 mg cholesterol; 0,3 g fibre
Exchanges: 1 starch; 1/2 meat; 2 fat

BAKED APRICOT PUDDING

75 g (150 ml) wholewheat flour, sifted and husks replaced
75 g (150 ml) flour, sifted
15 ml baking-powder
1 ml salt
4 ml liquid artificial sweetener
200 ml skim milk
25 g margarine, melted
410 g can unsweetened apricot halves in fruit juice, drained and juice reserved

Sift together flours, baking-powder and salt into a mixing-bowl. Add sweetener and milk. Pour melted margarine into a 1,25-litre ovenproof baking dish, swirl around to coat sides. Pour in batter, arrange apricot halves attractively on top. Bake at 180 °C, 45 to 50 minutes, until risen and firm.
Warm reserved juice, pour over pudding as soon as it comes out of the oven. Serve hot, with Diabetic Custard (see Pg 89).

Serves eight

Per serving: 448kJ; 16,3 g carbohydrate; 3,2 g protein; 2,9 g fat; 1 mg cholesterol; 1,7 g fibre
Exchanges: 1/2 fruit; 1 starch; 1/2 fat

PEACH CHEESECAKE

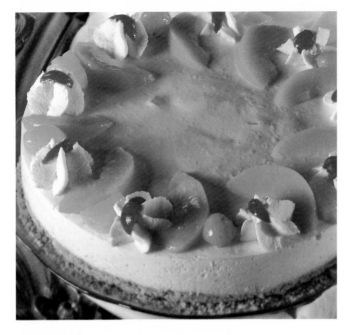

QUEEN OF PUDDINGS

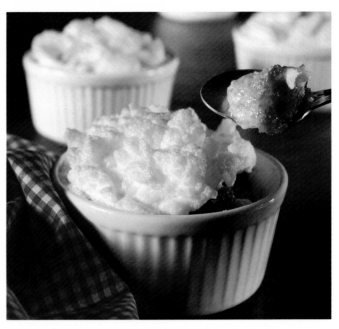

Crust
125 g cream cracker biscuits, crushed
1 ml liquid artificial sweetener
50 g margarine, melted

Filling
250 ml low-fat plain yoghurt
250 g tub low-fat smooth cottage cheese
**410 g can unsweetened fruit cocktail *or* peach slices,
   in their own juice**
5 ml liquid artificial sweetener
10 g (15 ml) gelatine, soaked in
50 ml reserved fruit juice
2 egg-whites, whipped

To decorate
Cream Substitute (see Pg 90)

Crust
Combine all ingredients in a bowl, stir well. Press on
to base of a lightly greased, 200 mm-diameter loose-
bottomed or springform pan, using the back of a metal
spoon. Chill well.

Filling
Beat together yoghurt and cottage cheese until smooth.
Chop half drained fruit roughly, stir into cheese mixture
with sweetener. Reserve juice.
Dissolve soaked gelatine over a saucepan of simmering
water, or in the microwave oven. Allow to cool, stir into
cheese mixture. Fold in whipped egg-whites, pour over
prepared crust, level surface. Cover lightly, chill in
refrigerator, at least four hours or overnight, until firm.
Carefully remove from pan, place on serving plate.
Decorate with rosettes of Cream Substitute and
remaining half of canned fruit. Brush fruit lightly with
reserved juice to moisten before serving.

Serves 12

5 thin slices wholewheat bread, crusts removed
8 ml finely grated lemon rind
20 g margarine, melted
10 ml liquid artificial sweetener
750 ml skim milk
2 eggs, separated
5 ml vanilla essence
80 g (60 ml) diabetic raspberry jam (spread)

Cut bread into 20 mm cubes. Combine with lemon rind,
toss well. Turn out on a lightly greased baking tray,
drizzle melted margarine over cubes, toss to coat.
Spread out into a single layer, bake at 200 °C,
10 minutes, or until crisp. Combine 5 ml sweetener,
milk, egg-yolks and vanilla essence in a saucepan.
Heat five minutes until warm but not thick.
Coat inside of six 180 ml soufflé dishes with non-stick
spray. Place about 80 ml bread cubes in each, top each
with 125 ml warmed custard. Stand in *bain marie*, so that
water reaches about 25 mm up sides of dishes. Bake at
180 °C, one hour. Pour off water from *bain marie*.
Warm diabetic jam, spread over each pudding. Whip
egg-whites with remaining 5 ml sweetener until stiff,
pile on to puddings. Return to oven a further 10 minutes
until lightly browned. Serve warm.

Serves six

Per serving: 707kJ; 25,4 g carbohydrate; 7,8 g protein; 4,2 g fat;
45 mg cholesterol; 1,9 g fibre
Exchanges: 1/2 skim milk; 1 starch; 1/2 fat

◄ Per serving: 520kJ; 12,3 g carbohydrate; 5,9 g protein; 5,8 g fat;
7 mg cholesterol; 0,5 g fibre
Exchanges: 1/2 starch; 1/2 meat; 1 fat

GRANADILLA CREAM

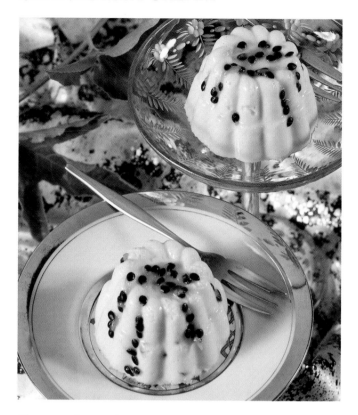

Use canned granadilla pulp if fresh fruit is not available; but rinse thoroughly to remove all sugar syrup.

500 ml skim milk
1 egg, separated
12 g (20 ml) gelatine
125 ml water
3 ml liquid artificial sweetener *or* to taste
5 ml vanilla essence
pulp of 2-3 granadillas

Per serving: 380kJ; 7,5 g carbohydrate; 9 g protein; 1,8 g fat; 62 mg cholesterol; 2,5 g fibre   Exchanges: 1/2 skim milk

Step 1:

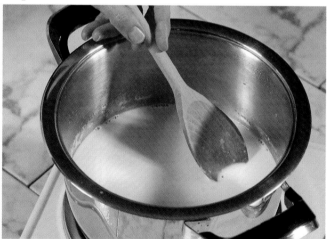

Heat milk and egg-yolk over medium heat, stirring continuously, until custard coats the back of a wooden spoon, about 10 minutes.

Step 2:

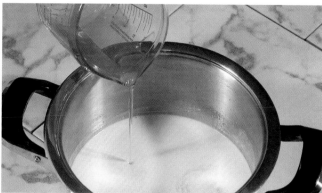

Soak gelatine in 50 ml of the water, dissolve over a saucepan of simmering water, or in microwave oven. Add remaining water, stir well, allow to cool. Add to custard, with sweetener and vanilla essence. Chill until beginning to thicken.

Step 3:

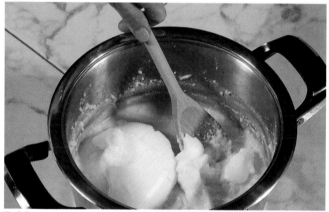

Fold in stiffly whipped egg-white.

Step 4:

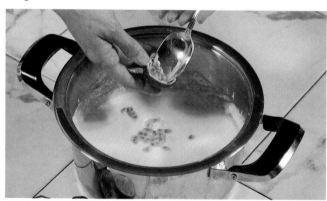

Fold in granadilla pulp.

To complete
Pour into four wetted, individual moulds, refrigerate until firm, three to four hours. Turn out on to small serving plates, decorate with extra granadilla pulp, if desired.

Serves four

VANILLA ICE-CREAM

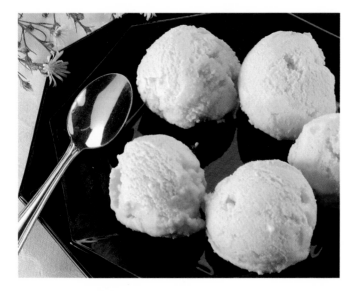

10 g (15 ml) gelatine
310 ml skim milk
2 eggs, separated
1 ml salt
5 ml liquid artificial sweetener
10 ml vanilla essence
half x 410 g can unsweetened evaporated milk, chilled
  overnight

Soak gelatine in 60 ml of the milk, dissolve over a
saucepan of simmering water, or in the microwave oven
on 100% (High) power, about 30 seconds. Set aside to
cool. Place remaining milk, egg-yolks, salt and
sweetener in the top of a double-boiler, whisk until
custard coats the back of wooden spoon. Add gelatine,
remove from heat, cool. Chill over ice until beginning to
thicken. Fold in vanilla essence and stiffly whipped
evaporated milk. Pour into suitable freezer container,
freeze four hours. Turn into a mixing-bowl, beat well to
break down ice-crystals. Fold in stiffly whipped egg-
whites. Return to freezer, freeze until firm, for 12 to
24 hours.

Makes about one litre, or four servings

Variations
Coffee flavour: Add 25 ml instant coffee powder dissolved
in 25 ml boiling water.
Caramel flavour: Substitute vanilla essence with 10 ml
caramel essence.
Orange flavour: Substitute vanilla essence with 10 ml
orange essence.
Chocolate flavour: Add 37,5 ml cocoa-powder dissolved in
37,5 ml boiling water.

Per serving: 799kJ; 15,1 g carbohydrate; 16,4 g protein; 6,7 g fat;
119 mg cholesterol; 0 g fibre
Exchanges: 1 whole milk

APPLE TRIANGLES

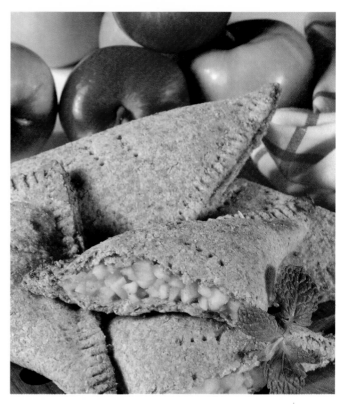

one quantity Wholewheat Pastry (see Pg 102)

Filling
2 large cooking apples, peeled, cored and chopped
juice and finely grated rind of half a lemon
little water
5 ml ground mixed spice
5 ml ground cinnamon
50 g (125 ml) mixed nuts, chopped
2 ml liquid artificial sweetener *or* to taste

Prepare pastry, wrap in clingwrap and refrigerate for
30 minutes.

Filling
Cook apples with lemon juice and rind in very little
water, until soft but not mushy, about 10 minutes.
Remove from heat, drain off any liquid. Combine with
rest of ingredients, set aside.
Roll out pastry thinly on a lightly floured surface, cut
into six equal squares. Divide filling between squares,
dampen edges and fold over to form large triangles.
Prick with a fork. Arrange on a lightly greased baking
tray, bake at 220 °C, 20 to 25 minutes. Serve hot, with
Diabetic Custard (see Pg 89).

Serves six

Per triangle: 334kJ; 8,4 g carbohydrate; 1,7 g protein; 4,6 g fat; 0 mg
cholesterol; 1,7 g fibre
Exchanges: 1 1/2 starch; 3 fat

BANANA AND DATE PUDDING

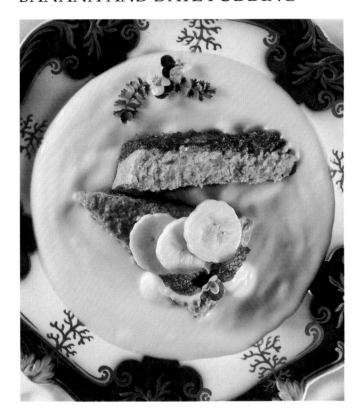

125 g (210 ml) pitted dates, chopped
juice of one large lemon
50 ml water
3 ripe bananas
125 g (350 ml) rolled oats
1 extra-large egg, beaten
200 ml skim milk
10 ml ground mixed spice
finely grated rind of half a lemon
1 ml liquid artificial sweetener *or* to taste

Place dates, lemon juice and water in a saucepan. Cook gently, five minutes. Remove from heat, spread over base of a lightly greased 750 ml ovenproof dish. Mash two bananas, combine with oats, egg and milk. Add spice, lemon rind and sweetener to taste, spread over dates. Bake at 180 °C, 25 to 30 minutes. Remove from oven, top with third banana, sliced, for decoration. Serve at once, with Diabetic Custard (see Pg 89).

Serves eight

STRAWBERRY-PINEAPPLE CHEESECAKE

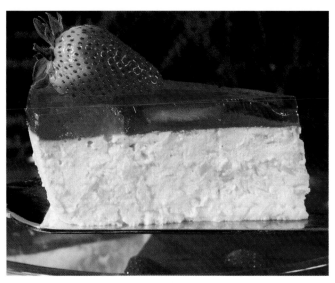

3 x 250 g tubs low-fat smooth cottage cheese
425 g can unsweetened pineapple rings in fruit juice, undrained, chopped
20 g (30 ml) gelatine, soaked in 125 ml water
8 ml liquid artificial sweetener *or* to taste
10 ml vanilla essence
125 ml skim milk

Topping
10 g sachet diabetic jelly-powder (strawberry flavour)
125 g fresh strawberries, washed, hulled and halved
few whole strawberries for decoration

Place cottage cheese and can of pineapples with juice in bowl of electric blender or food processor. Dissolve soaked gelatine over a saucepan of simmering water, or in microwave oven. Cool slightly, add to cheese mixture with sweetener, vanilla essence and milk. Blend until smooth. Pour into a lightly greased, deep 230 mm-square or round pie-dish. Chill in refrigerator until firm. Meanwhile, make up jelly according to instructions on box, allow to cool. Chill over ice until just beginning to thicken. Arrange strawberry halves attractively over cheesecake, spoon thickened jelly carefully over surface. Return to refrigerator until firm.

Serves 12

Per serving: 671kJ; 29 g carbohydrate; 4,1 g protein; 2,8 g fat; 30 mg cholesterol; 3.3 g fibre
Exchanges: 1 fruit; 1/2 starch

Per serving: 372kJ; 5,3 g carbohydrate; 10 g protein; 2,8 g fat; 9 mg cholesterol; 0,5 g fibre
Exchanges: 1/2 fruit; 1 meat

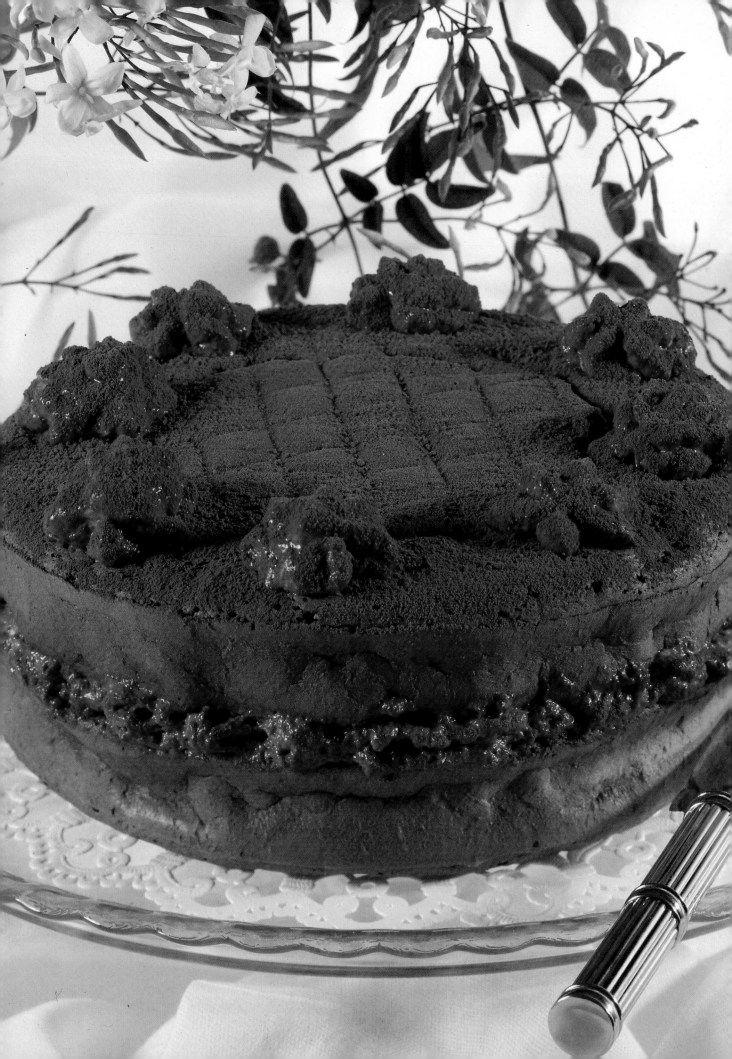

BAKING

These diabetic bakes have been made healthier by using fibre-rich wholewheat flour, less fat, and artificial sweetener. Include a slice of bread or roll in your daily diet, but regard cakes and cookies as treats, to be eaten only on the odd occasion, or for a special celebration.
Bakes made with artificial sweetener do not have the keeping quality of those made with sugar, and should be eaten the day they're prepared. Some may be stored overnight in the refrigerator, or frozen for up to three months. Make toppings, frostings and fillings just before serving – they don't keep or freeze.
Using wholewheat flour, particularly in cakes and biscuits, results in a heavy, close texture. To alleviate this, plain white or self-raising flour has been combined with the wholewheat flour for a much lighter end-product. Texture will also be greatly improved by sifting the dry ingredients several times.

WHOLEWHEAT CHOCOLATE APPLE CAKE

125 g (250 ml) wholewheat flour, sifted and husks
  replaced
125 g (250 ml) flour, sifted
30 g (75 ml) cocoa-powder, sifted
15 ml baking-powder
2 ml salt
10 ml liquid artificial sweetener
5 egg-whites
160 ml bottled unsweetened apple sauce
625 ml skim milk
5 ml vanilla essence

To decorate
one quantity Cream Substitute (see Pg 90)
10 g (25 ml) cocoa-powder, dissolved in
25 ml boiling water
10 g (25 ml) cocoa-powder, sifted, extra

Sift together dry ingredients into a mixing-bowl. Place sweetener, egg-whites and apple sauce in mixer-bowl, beat on high speed, two minutes. Add milk and vanilla essence to flour mixture, beat lightly. Add to egg-white mixture, fold in. Pour batter into two greased and lined 200 mm-diameter sandwich pans. Bake at 180 °C, 30 to 40 minutes. Turn out on to wire cooling racks, allow to cool completely.
Make up Cream Substitute as in recipe, adding dissolved cocoa-powder with gelatine to the heated milk. When stiff, use two-thirds to sandwich layers together, and remainder to pipe rosettes on top. (Diabetic jam or apple sauce may be used as filling, if

preferred.) Dust top of cake with extra sifted cocoa-powder and serve at once.

Serves eight to 10

(Based on eight servings) Per serving: 860kJ; 26,9 g carbohydrate; 12,1 g protein; 4,6 g fat; 13 mg cholesterol; 2,8 g fibre
Exchanges: 1 1/2 starch

DIABETIC CUP-CAKES

This batter may also be divided between two 150 mm-diameter sandwich cake pans. Bake at 190 °C, about 15 minutes. Sandwich together with diabetic jam.

2 extra-large eggs, separated
4 ml liquid artificial sweetener
1 ml vanilla essence
60 g (125 ml) bran-rich self-raising flour, sifted and
  husks replaced
pinch of salt

Whisk egg-whites until stiff peaks form, add egg-yolks one at a time, beating well after each. Add sweetener and vanilla essence, beat until mixture is thick and pale. Fold in sifted flour and salt. Spoon into 12 lightly greased or paper-case-lined patty pans. Bake at 180 °C, 15 minutes. Remove to wire cooling rack to cool. Serve plain, or top with diabetic jam.

Makes 12

(Without jam) Per two cup-cakes: 256kJ; 6,2 g carbohydrate; 3,6 g protein; 2 g fat; 76 mg cholesterol; 1,2 g fibre
Exchanges: 1/2 starch

◄ Wholewheat chocolate apple cake

FROSTED CHOCOLATE SQUARES

If bran-rich self-raising flour is not available, use wholewheat flour with 10 ml baking-powder.

Cake
190 g (375 ml) bran-rich self-raising flour, sifted and husks replaced
9 ml liquid artificial sweetener
50 g (125 ml) cocoa-powder
3 ml bicarbonate of soda
2 ml salt
250 ml skim milk
100 ml cooking oil
2 large eggs, beaten

Chocolate frosting
250 ml skim milk
12 g (25 ml) cornflour
8 ml liquid artificial sweetener
25 g (60 ml) cocoa-powder
5 ml vanilla essence
pinch of salt
37,5 ml water

Cake
Combine all ingredients in a mixer-bowl, beat just until blended. Pour into a greased and lined 230 mm by 330 mm baking tray, level surface. Bake at 180 °C, about 20 minutes, or until firm. Remove from oven, set aside.

Chocolate frosting
Combine all ingredients in a saucepan. Cook over medium heat, stirring continuously, until thick. Allow to cool, beat well until of a spreading consistency. Spread frosting over cake, cut into squares. Best eaten the same day, or store, covered, in refrigerator overnight.

Makes 45 squares

Per square: 188kJ; 3,2 g carbohydrate; 1,6 g protein; 2,7 g fat; 8 mg cholesterol; 0,7 g fibre
Exchanges: 1 starch; 1 fat

WHOLEWHEAT YOGHURT SCONES

150 g (300 ml) wholewheat flour, sifted and husks replaced
5 ml baking-powder
1 ml bicarbonate of soda
pinch of salt
30 g margarine
175 ml carton low-fat plain yoghurt

Combine flour, baking-powder, bicarbonate of soda and salt in a mixing-bowl. Rub in margarine until mixture resembles fine crumbs. Add yoghurt, stir to form a soft

dough. Turn out on to a well-floured surface, pat out to about 20 mm-thickness. Cut into eight squares. Place on a lightly greased baking tray, bake at 190 °C, 15 to 20 minutes, until well risen and golden brown. Serve with margarine and diabetic jam.

Makes eight

(Without margarine or jam) Per scone: 407kJ; 11,1 g carbohydrate; 3,4 g protein; 4 g fat; 1 mg cholesterol; 2 g fibre
Exchanges: 1 starch; 1 1/2 fat

OAT AND RAISIN COOKIES

150 g (300 ml) wholewheat flour, sifted and husks replaced
pinch of salt
2 ml baking-powder
1 ml bicarbonate of soda
2 ml ground cinnamon
1 ml ground nutmeg
60 g (100 ml) seedless raisins, chopped
200 g (550 ml) rolled oats
10 ml liquid artificial sweetener
60 g margarine, melted
1 small egg, beaten
125 ml skim milk

Sift together dry ingredients into a mixing-bowl. Stir in raisins and oats. Combine remaining ingredients, add to dry ingredients, stir well to bind. Using hands, shape into 35 small balls, place on lightly greased baking trays. Flatten each slightly with a fork. Bake at 190 °C, about 25 minutes, until golden brown. Remove to wire cooling rack and allow to cool. Store in an airtight container.

Makes 35

Per three cookies: 740kJ; 22,5 g carbohydrate; 4,6 g protein; 6,5 g fat; 17 mg cholesterol; 3,6 g fibre
Exchanges: 1 starch; 1 fat

Clockwise from back right: Frosted chocolate squares; Wholewheat yoghurt scones; Oat and raisin cookies ➤

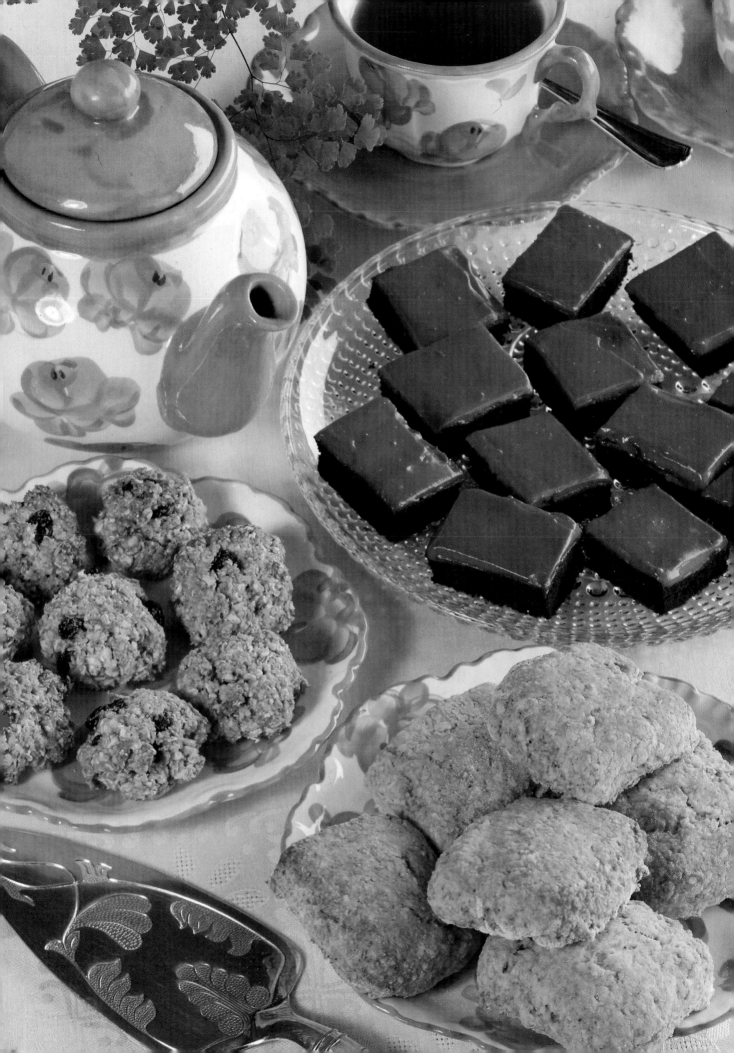

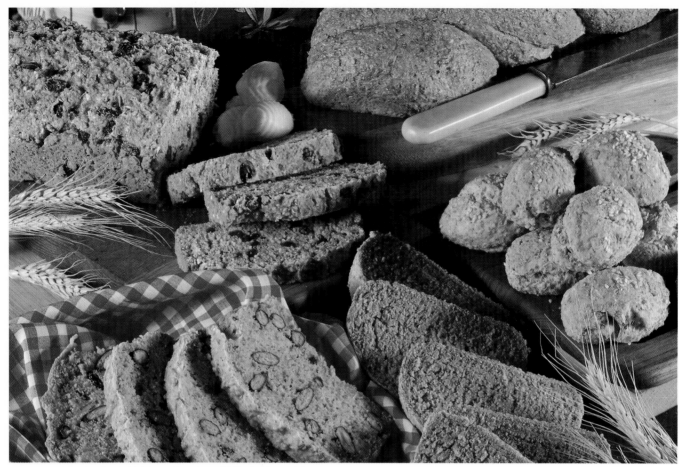

Clockwise from back left: Raisin and oat bread; Wholewheat plait; Wholewheat potato rolls; Granary loaf; Wholewheat bean and cheese loaf

RAISIN AND OAT BREAD

Bran-rich self-raising flour may be substituted for half self-raising flour, half wholewheat flour, and 10 ml baking-powder, if preferred.

350 g (700 ml) bran-rich self-raising flour, sifted and
   husks replaced
120 g (250 ml) rolled oats
5 ml salt
100 g (165 ml) seedless raisins
10 ml ground mixed spice
2 ml liquid artificial sweetener
350 ml low-fat plain yoghurt
50 ml water

Combine flour, oats, salt, raisins and spice in a mixing-bowl. In a separate jug, mix together sweetener, yoghurt and water, add to dry ingredients to form a soft dough. Shape into an oblong, drop into a lightly greased 500 g loaf pan, bake at 200 °C, about 45 minutes. Turn out on to a wire cooling rack to cool. Serve sliced and spread with margarine.

Makes one loaf, or 12 to 15 slices

(Based on 12 slices, without margarine) Per slice: 783kJ; 34,8 g carbohydrate; 5,8 g protein; 1,8 g fat; 2 mg cholesterol; 2,2 g fibre
Exchanges: 1 1/2 starch

WHOLEWHEAT PLAIT

250 ml skim milk
300 ml lukewarm water
25 g cube fresh yeast *or* 15 ml dried yeast
500 g (4 x 250 ml) wholewheat flour, sifted and husks
   replaced
100 g (125 ml) crushed wheat
150 g (300 ml) white bread flour, sifted
10 ml salt
30 g margarine
1 egg-white, lightly frothed

Add milk to water, stir to combine. Blend yeast with 150 ml of the liquid, cover and leave in a warm, draught-free place until frothy, about 15 minutes. Combine dry ingredients in a large mixing-bowl. Stir margarine into remaining lukewarm liquid, allow to melt. Make a well in centre of dry ingredients, pour in yeast mixture and remaining liquid, mix to form a firm dough, adding more water if necessary. Turn out on to a lightly floured surface, knead well 10 minutes.
Place dough in a lightly oiled bowl, cover with clingwrap and a dampened tea-towel, leave in a warm, draught-free place, until doubled in bulk, for about two hours.
Knock back, divide in half. Form each into a long sausage, join ends. Plait loosely, join other end. Place on a greased and floured baking tray. Brush dough lightly

with oil, cover and leave to rise until doubled in bulk, about 45 minutes. Brush with egg-white, bake at 220 °C, 30 to 35 minutes. Check after 20 minutes – reduce temperature if bread is browning too quickly. Remove to a wire cooling rack to cool completely.

Makes one large loaf (about 30 slices), or 24 rolls.

(Based on 30 slices) Per slice: 476kJ; 19,4 g carbohydrate; 4,3 g protein; 1,1 g fat; 0 mg cholesterol; 3,4 g fibre
Exchanges: 1 starch

WHOLEWHEAT POTATO ROLLS

Use half wholewheat flour, half self-raising flour, and 5 ml baking-powder, instead of the bran-rich self-raising flour, if preferred.

180 g (360 ml) bran-rich self-raising flour, sifted and husks replaced
90 g potato, cooked, skinned and mashed
1 egg, lightly beaten
150 ml skim milk
sesame seeds to sprinkle

Combine flour, potato and egg in a mixing-bowl. Gradually add milk to form a smooth dough. Divide into nine equal pieces, form into rolls. Place on a lightly greased baking tray. Bake at 200 °C, 25 to 30 minutes, until golden brown. Remove to a wire cooling rack to cool completely.

Makes nine rolls

Per roll: 420kJ; 17,2 g carbohydrate; 3,9 g protein; 1,3 g fat; 25 mg cholesterol; 0,7 g fibre
Exchanges: 1 starch

GRANARY LOAF

Stone-ground flour, containing all the components of wholewheat, including bran, wheatgerm and gluten, is available in 1 kg cloth bags from various kitchen speciality shops and farmstalls in the Cape, Natal, and Transvaal; or direct from the Josephine Mill in Cape Town. Stone-ground flour may be used instead of wholewheat flour in any of the baking recipes given here – the texture will be denser, though.

425 g (850 ml) stone-ground flour, sifted
200 g (400 ml) white bread flour, sifted
10 ml salt
25 g cube fresh yeast *or* 15 ml dried yeast
about 350 ml lukewarm water

Sift together dry ingredients into a large mixing-bowl. Mix yeast with 125 ml of the water, cover and leave in a warm, draught-free place until frothy, about 15 minutes. Add to dry ingredients, with enough remaining luke-

warm water to form a firm dough. Knead until smooth. Place dough in a lightly oiled bowl, cover with cling-wrap and dampened tea-towel, leave in a warm, draught-free place until doubled in bulk, for about one hour.
Knock down, knead three to four minutes. Pat out into a rectangle, roll up like a Swiss-roll. Cut three diagonal cuts across top of roll. Place on a lightly greased baking tray. Cover and leave in a warm place until doubled in bulk, about 30 minutes.
Bake at 220 °C, 20 minutes. Reduce heat to 190 °C, bake a further 10 minutes, or until bread sounds hollow when rapped underneath with the knuckles. Remove to a wire cooling rack to cool.

Makes one loaf, or about 15 slices

(Based on 15 slices) Per slice: 643kJ; 31,6 g carbohydrate; 3,9 g protein; 0,4 g fat; 0 mg cholesterol; 1,4 g fibre
Exchanges: 2 starch

WHOLEWHEAT BEAN AND CHEESE LOAF

Substitute bran-rich self-raising flour for 200 g (400 ml) wholewheat flour, 75 g (150 ml) white flour, and 10 ml baking-powder, if preferred.

60 g margarine
275 g (550 ml) bran-rich self-raising flour, sifted
3 ml salt
5 ml dry mustard powder
5 ml baking-powder
5 ml dried mixed herbs
90 g (225 ml) low-fat hard cheese, grated
425 g can red kidney beans, drained and rinsed
150 ml skim milk
1 egg, beaten

Rub margarine into sifted flour and salt. Add mustard, baking-powder, herbs, cheese and beans, stir well. Combine milk and egg, stir into mixture until a soft dough is formed. Turn into a lightly greased 500 g loaf pan. Bake at 180 °C, one hour, until well risen and golden brown. Leave to cool in pan 10 minutes, before turning out on to a wire cooling rack to cool completely. Serve, cut in slices and spread with margarine.

Makes one loaf, or 12 to 15 slices

(Based on 12 slices) Per slice: 1 100kJ; 32 g carbohydrate; 13,9 g protein; 6,4 g fat; 24 mg cholesterol; 8,3 g fibre
Exchanges: 1 1/2 starch; 1/2 meat; 1 fat

SPICY BRAN MUFFINS

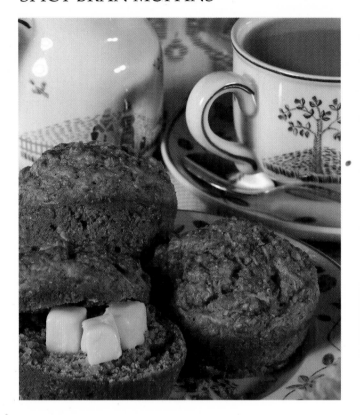

30 g (60 ml) skim milk powder
15 ml baking-powder
3 ml salt
10 ml ground mixed spice
70 g (350 ml) lightly crushed All-bran flakes
155 g (310 ml) wholewheat flour, sifted and husks
  replaced
10 ml finely grated orange rind
2 eggs, beaten
5 ml liquid artificial sweetener
5 ml cooking oil
250 ml skim milk
200 ml grated apple
1 small carrot, scraped and grated

Combine milk powder, baking-powder, salt, spice, flakes, flour and orange rind in a mixing-bowl. Beat together eggs, sweetener, oil and milk, pour into dry ingredients, stir well. Add apple and carrot, blend lightly. Fill greased muffin pans two-thirds with mixture, bake at 200 °C, about 25 minutes until well risen and firm. Serve plain, or halved and spread with margarine.

Makes 15

(Without margarine) Per muffin: 284kJ; 9,8 g carbohydrate; 3,7 g protein; 1 g fat; 29 mg cholesterol; 3,3 g fibre
Exchanges: 1/2 starch

DIABETIC COOKIE-PRESS BISCUITS

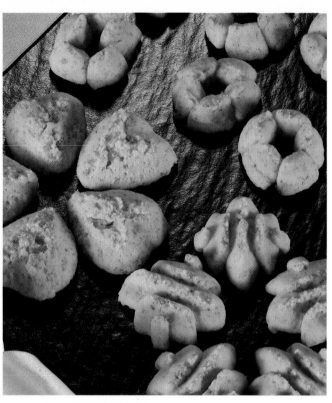

Vary the flavour by adding essence, or grated citrus rind to the basic recipe. Not suitable for those on a weight-reducing diet, due to the high fat content.

250 g margarine
7 ml liquid artificial sweetener *or* to taste
2 extra-large eggs, beaten
60 g (125 ml) bran-rich self-raising flour, sifted
190 g (375 ml) flour, sifted
60 g (125 ml) cornflour, sifted

Cream together margarine and sweetener, beat in eggs. Sift together dry ingredients, add to creamed mixture. Mix to form a firm but pliable dough. Press through cookie-maker on to lightly greased baking trays, bake at 200 °C, about 15 minutes, or until pale golden brown. Remove to wire cooling rack to cool completely. Store in airtight container.

Makes about 70

Per three biscuits: 459kJ; 11,4 g carbohydrate; 1,5 g protein; 6 g fat; 12 mg cholesterol; 0,6 g fibre
Exchanges: 1/2 starch; 2 fat

SUGAR-FREE CARROT CAKE

Bran-rich self-raising flour may be substituded for half wholewheat flour, half self-raising flour, and 5 ml baking-powder, if desired.

250 g (500 ml) bran-rich self-raising flour, sifted and husks replaced
10 ml baking-powder
10 ml ground cinnamon
2 ml salt
8 ml liquid artificial sweetener
250 g carrots, scraped and grated
juice and finely grated rind of one large orange
3 extra-large eggs, beaten
125 ml sunflower oil

Cream cheese icing
250 g tub low-fat smooth cottage cheese
finely grated rind of half an orange
4 drops liquid artificial sweetener
5 ml gelatine, soaked in
25 ml fresh orange juice

To decorate
thin slivers of orange rind
walnut halves (optional)

Combine dry ingredients in a mixing-bowl. Add sweetener, carrots, orange juice and rind. Beat together eggs and oil, add to batter, stir well to blend. Pour batter into a lightly greased, two-litre tube-pan, bake at 190 °C, 40 to 45 minutes, or until a skewer inserted into the centre comes out clean. Remove from oven, leave to stand five minutes. Turn out on to a wire cooling rack, allow to cool completely.

Cream cheese icing
Empty cheese into a small bowl, beat well. Add orange rind and sweetener, stir to blend. Dissolve soaked gelatine over a saucepan of simmering water, or in microwave oven on 100% (High) power, 20 to 30 seconds. Allow to cool. Add to cheese mixture, stir well. Refrigerate until slightly thickened.

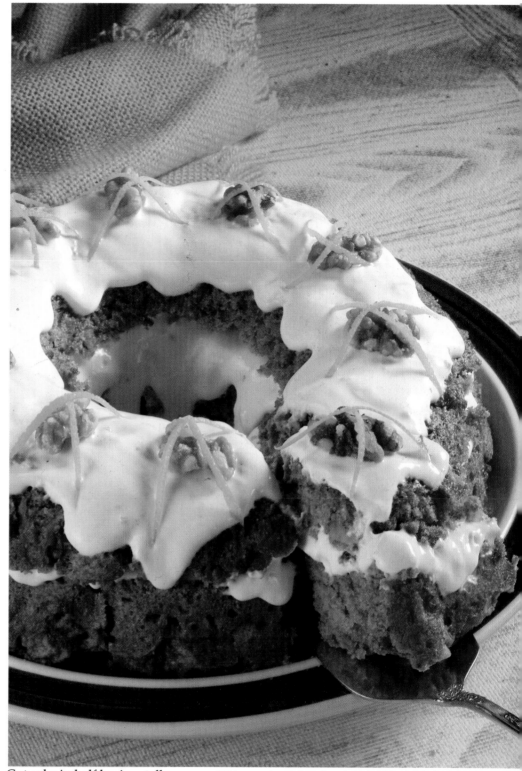

Cut cake in half horizontally, sandwich together with Cream Cheese Icing. Spread remaining icing over the top of the cake, allowing it to run down sides slightly. Decorate with thin slivers of orange rind and walnut halves, if desired.

Makes 16 slices

(Without walnuts) Per slice: 647kJ; 12,3 g carbohydrate; 4,5 g protein; 9 g fat; 2 mg cholesterol; 2,8 g fibre
Exchanges: 1 starch; 1/2 meat; 1 1/2 fat

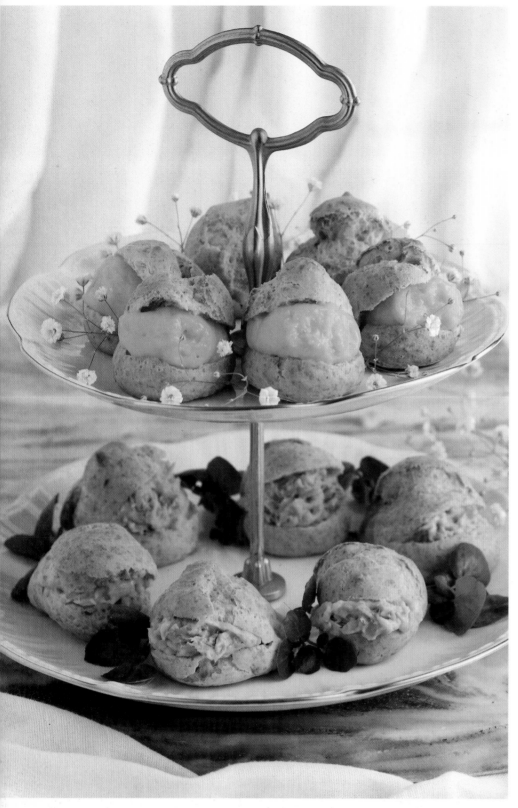

WHOLEWHEAT CHOUX PUFFS

Choux pastry
150 ml water
40 g margarine
1 ml salt
38 g (75 ml) wholewheat flour,
  sifted and husks replaced
38 g (75 ml) flour, sifted
4 drops liquid artificial
  sweetener (optional)
2 eggs

Suggested fillings
thick Diabetic Custard
  (see recipe on Pg 89)
tuna in a thick white sauce
  (see recipe on Pg 92)

Choux pastry
Bring water and margarine to
the boil in a small saucepan.
Remove from heat, add
combined salt and flours *all at
once*, beat well with a wooden
spoon. Add sweetener and one
egg, beat well by hand until
mixture is smooth. Add second
egg, a little at a time, until
pastry is smooth, shiny and of a
piping consistency.
Don't make it too soft.
Fill a piping bag fitted with a
large, plain nozzle, with pastry.
Pipe blobs on to a lightly
greased baking tray, cutting off
dough each time with a small,
sharp knife. Bake at 200 °C,
25 to 30 minutes, until well
risen, crisp and golden brown.
Remove from oven, cut a small
horizontal slit in centre of each
one to allow steam to escape.
Place on a wire cooling rack
to cool.
Pipe or spoon sweet or savoury
filling into puffs, serve within
30 minutes of completion.
Serve with afternoon tea; as a
pre-dinner snack; as a dessert;
or as a light meal with salad.

Makes 12

*Freeze unfilled, baked puffs in rigid containers, with foil between layers. Store for up
to six months. Reheat from frozen at 190 °C for seven to 10 minutes. Any number of
sweet or savoury fillings may be used – see recipe for Open Sandwiches (Pg 60) for
savoury suggestions. Sweet fillings include sweetened yoghurt, flavoured cottage
cheese, thick custard, fruit or diabetic jam.*

Per puff: 190kJ; 1,9 g carbohydrate;
1,5 g protein; 3,4 g fat;
38 mg cholesterol; 0,4 g fibre
Exchanges: 1/2 starch; 1/2 fat

SWEET FRUIT TARTLETS

If preferred, use the wholewheat shortcrust pastry from the Cornish Pasties, Pg 62, instead of the potato pastry given here.

Potato pastry
125 g (250 ml) wholewheat flour, sifted and husks replaced
125 g (250 ml) flour, sifted
pinch of salt
80 g margarine
100 g potato, cooked, skinned and mashed
12,5 ml water

Filling
200 g low-fat smooth cottage cheese
variety of fresh fruit in season *or* canned unsweetened fruit in fruit juice, drained
300 ml prepared diabetic jelly, in various colours

Potato pastry
Sift together flours and salt. Rub in margarine. Stir in mashed potato, knead with water until firm. Roll out thinly on a lightly floured surface, cut into 20 mm by 80 mm-diameter rounds. Line lightly greased patty pans with pastry, prick well with a fork. Bake at 200 °C, 15 minutes. Remove from oven, leave in pans to cool.

Filling
Divide cottage cheese between tartlet cases, smooth over with a teaspoon. Arrange pieces of fruit on cheese. Leave jelly to cool. Stand over ice until beginning to thicken. Spoon about 12,5 ml slightly thickened jelly carefully over fruit, covering completely.
Refrigerate until firm, about one hour, or until ready to serve.

Makes 20

Per tartlet: 357kJ; 9,3 g carbohydrate; 2,7 g protein; 4 g fat; 2 mg cholesterol; 1,1 g fibre
Exchanges: 1/2 starch; 1 fat

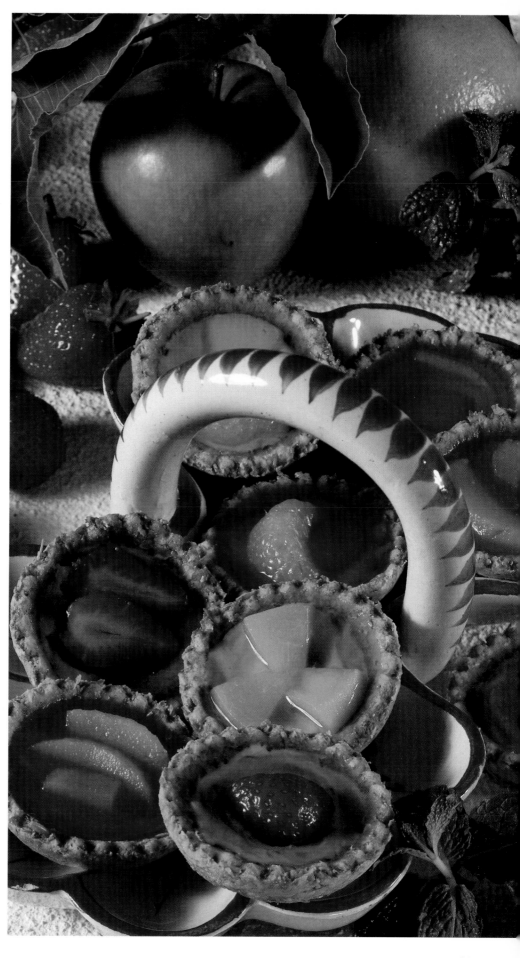

VANILLA SANDWICH CAKE WITH CREAMY FROSTING

Use this frosting for the Christmas cake, if preferred (see Pg 104). May also be used instead of jam, to sandwich together cakes and biscuits.

Sandwich cake
90 g margarine
2 eggs, beaten
1 egg-white
125 g (250 ml) wholewheat flour, sifted and husks replaced
100 g (200 ml) flour, sifted
12,5 ml baking-powder
pinch of salt
150 ml skim milk
5 ml vanilla essence
5 ml liquid artificial sweetener

Creamy frosting
125 g low-fat smooth cottage cheese
1 ml salt
3 ml soft margarine
5 ml liquid artificial sweetener
2 ml flavouring essence (almond, vanilla *or* own choice)

Sandwich cake
Place margarine in a mixer-bowl. Add eggs and egg-white, beat well. Sift together flours, baking-powder and salt. In a separate bowl, combine milk, vanilla essence and sweetener. Add two mixtures alternately to egg mixture, beating continuously until combined.
Pour into two greased and base-lined 200 mm-diameter cake pans. Bake at 180 °C, 25 to 30 minutes, or until a skewer inserted into the centre comes out clean. Remove cakes from oven, leave in pans five minutes before turning out on to a wire cooling rack to cool.

Creamy frosting
Beat together all ingredients until light and smooth. Sandwich cake layers together with diabetic jam. Top with Creamy Frosting, and serve at once.

Serves 12

Per slice: 521kJ; 13 g carbohydrate; 4,3 g protein; 5,8 g fat; 23 mg cholesterol; 1,5 g fibre
Exchanges: 1 starch; 1/2 meat; 1 1/2 fat

CINNAMON BISCUITS

60 g (125 ml) flour, sifted
60 g (125 ml) wholewheat flour, sifted and husks replaced
3 ml baking-powder
60 g margarine
10 ml vanilla essence
5 ml liquid artificial sweetener
25 ml fresh orange juice
5 ml ground cinnamon

Sift together flours and baking-powder into a mixing-bowl. Rub in margarine. Stir in vanilla essence, sweetener and orange juice. Blend well to form a firm dough. Sprinkle with cinnamon, knead in lightly. Break off small pieces, roll into balls about 10 mm in diameter. Arrange on a lightly greased baking tray, flatten slightly with a fork. Bake at 180 °C, 15 to 18 minutes, until pale golden brown. Remove to a wire cooling rack to cool completely. Store in an airtight tin.

Makes 20

Per three biscuits: 558kJ; 12,6 g carbohydrate; 1,8 g protein; 8,1 g fat; 0 mg cholesterol; 1,5 g fibre
Exchanges: 1 starch; 2 fat

THIRTY-DAY HEALTH MUFFINS

Mixture may be kept in refrigerator for up to 30 days before using. Take out as much batter as you need, return remainder to refrigerator to ensure a steady supply of freshly baked muffins.

125 ml sunflower oil
2 extra-large eggs, beaten
625 ml skim milk
125 g (250 ml) wholewheat flour, sifted and husks replaced
190 g (375 ml) flour, sifted
80 g (500 ml) digestive bran
5 ml vanilla essence
5 ml salt
10 ml bicarbonate of soda
150 g (250 ml) stoned dates, chopped

Whisk together oil and eggs in a large mixing-bowl. Add remaining ingredients, blend well. Cover tightly, leave in refrigerator overnight.
Two-thirds fill lightly greased muffin pans with batter. Bake at 180 °C, 20 to 25 minutes, until well risen and springy to the touch. Remove to wire cooling racks to cool completely. Serve plain, or split and spread with margarine.

Makes 24 large muffins

(Without margarine) Per muffin: 547kJ; 15,5 g carbohydrate; 3,4 g protein; 5,9 g fat; 22 mg cholesterol; 2,4 g fibre
Exchanges: 1 starch; 1 fat

WHOLEWHEAT BANANA COOKIES

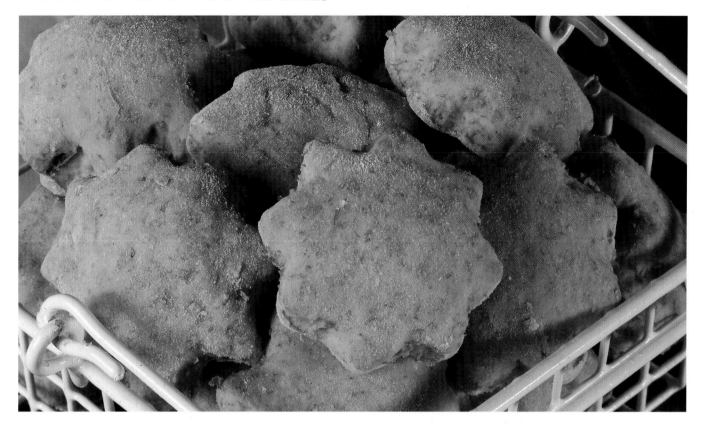

125 g (250 ml) flour, sifted
125 g (250 ml) wholewheat flour, sifted and husks
  replaced
10 ml baking-powder
1 ml bicarbonate of soda
2 ml ground cinnamon
pinch of ground nutmeg
40 g margarine
125 ml mashed banana (2 medium bananas)
60 ml low-fat plain yoghurt
2 ml liquid artificial sweetener *or* to taste
5 ml vanilla essence
37,5 ml skim milk

Sift together dry ingredients into a mixing-bowl. Rub in
margarine until mixture resembles fine breadcrumbs.
Add mashed banana. Combine yoghurt, sweetener,
vanilla essence and milk, mix into flour mixture until a
firm dough is formed.
Turn out dough on to a lightly floured surface, knead
well three to four minutes, adding more flour if dough
sticks to hands. Roll out to 10 mm-thickness, cut out
biscuits using a 50 mm-diameter biscuit cutter. Place on
a lightly greased baking tray, bake at 220 °C, 10 to
12 minutes until pale golden brown. Remove from oven,
leave on tray one to two minutes before removing to a
wire cooling rack to cool completely. Store in an
airtight tin.

Makes 36

Per two cookies: 656kJ; 25,8 g carbohydrate; 4,4 g protein; 3,4 g fat;
0 mg cholesterol; 2,6 g fibre
Exchanges: 1 1/2 starch; 1 fat

SUGARLESS BANANA BREAD

110 g (220 ml) wholewheat flour, sifted and husks
  replaced
110 g (220 ml) flour, sifted
12,5 ml baking-powder
1 ml bicarbonate of soda
3 ml salt
60 g margarine, melted
2 eggs, beaten
8 ml liquid artificial sweetener
5 ml vanilla essence
2 bananas, mashed

Sift together dry ingredients into a mixing-bowl. Stir in
next four ingredients, just enough to moisten mixture.
Mix in mashed bananas. Pour batter into a greased and
lined 500 g loaf pan. Bake at 180 °C, 45 to 50 minutes, or
until a skewer inserted into the centre comes out clean.
Turn out on to wire cooling rack, allow to cool
completely. Serve, thickly sliced and spread with
margarine.

Makes 16 slices

(Without margarine) Per slice: 450kJ; 13,3 g carbohydrate;
2,9 g protein; 4,5 g fat; 34 mg cholesterol; 1,4 g fibre
Exchanges: 1 starch; 1 fat

CRUNCHY HAZEL-NUT MOUNDS

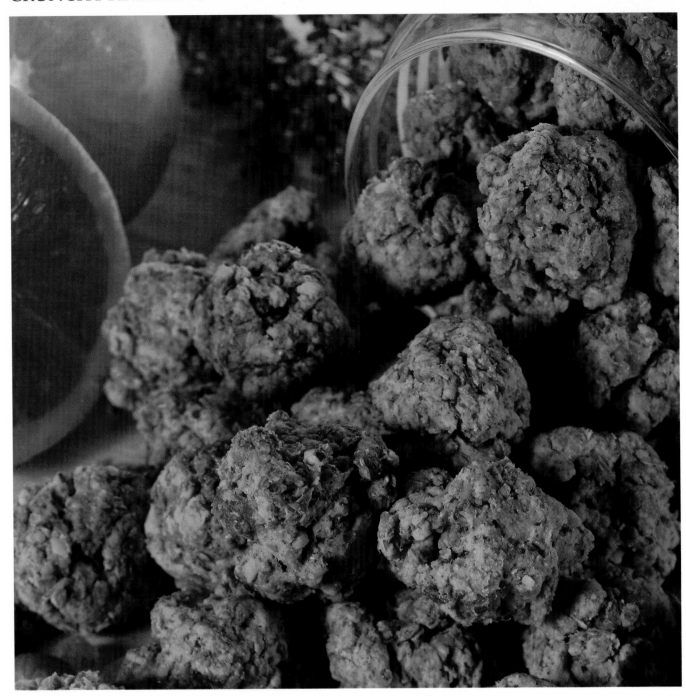

225 g (450 ml) wholewheat flour, sifted and husks
  replaced
30 g (125 ml) lightly crushed All-bran flakes
100 g (250 ml) hazel-nuts, coarsely ground
15 ml baking-powder
pinch of salt
60 g margarine
100 g potato, cooked, skinned and mashed
5 ml liquid artificial sweetener
60 g (100 ml) sultanas, roughly chopped
finely grated rind of one orange
10 ml ground mixed spice
1 egg, beaten
25 ml low-fat plain yoghurt

Per two biscuits: 350kJ; 7,8 g carbohydrate; 2,2 g protein; 4,6 g fat;
8 mg cholesterol; 2,2 g fibre
Exchanges: 1 starch; 1 fat

Step 1:

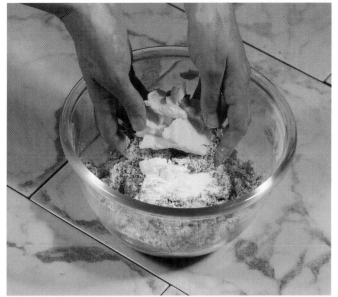

Combine flour, flakes, nuts, baking-powder and salt in a mixing-bowl. Rub in margarine.

Step 2:

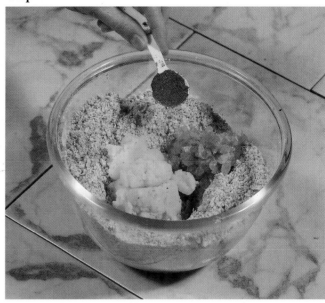

Beat together mashed potato and sweetener, add to flour mixture with sultanas, orange rind and spice.

Step 3:

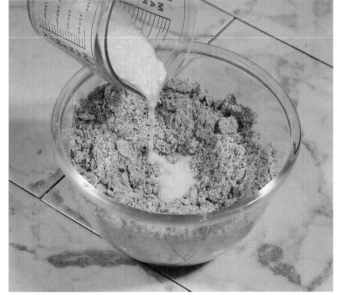

Beat together egg and yoghurt, add to dry ingredients, mixing well to form a stiff dough.

Step 4:

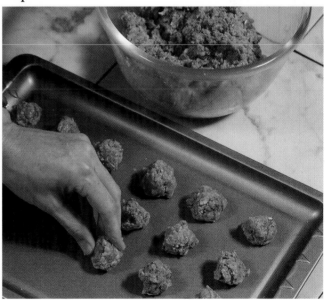

Using about 15 ml mixture at a time, form into small rough mounds on two large, lightly greased baking trays, pushing together with fingertips.

To complete
Bake at 200 °C, about 15 minutes, or until lightly browned and firm. Remove to wire cooling rack, allow to cool completely. Store in an airtight tin.

Makes about 50

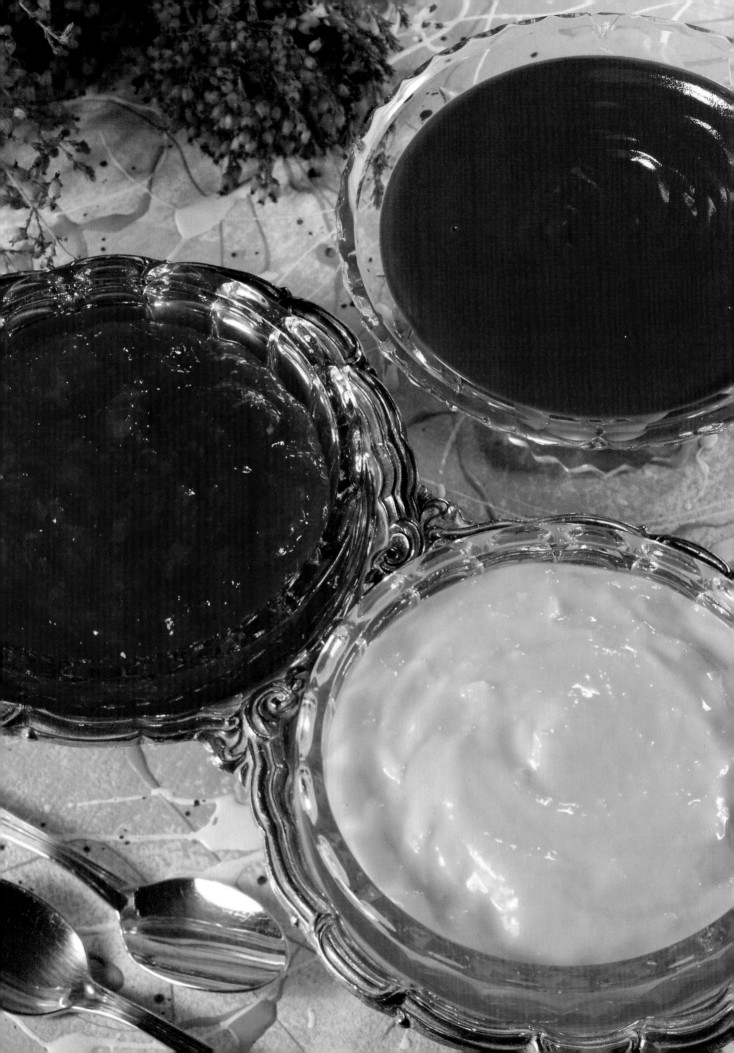

SAUCES AND DRESSINGS

Many commercial sauces contain sugar, making them taboo for diabetics. Always read the labels carefully and, when in doubt, don't buy. Rather make your own at home, when you can be sure ingredients used are within your dietetic allowances.
Included in this section are: savoury sauces, salad dressings, burger toppings, and accompanying sauces for meat, fish and vegetarian dishes; sweet sauces to add flavour and eye-appeal to that cool, refreshing ice-cream or warm, baked dessert; suggestions for creamy cake fillings and whipped toppings.

CHOCOLATE SAUCE

12 g (25 ml) cornflour
15 g (37,5 ml) cocoa-powder
75 ml water
450 ml skim milk
5 ml liquid artificial sweetener *or* to taste

Stir cornflour and cocoa into water, add to milk in a small saucepan. Bring to the boil, stirring all the time. Reduce heat, cook gently five minutes, stirring continuously, until thickened. Sweeten to taste. Serve hot, over ice-cream, or canned fruit.

Makes 375 ml, or 30 by 12,5 ml servings

(Based on 30 servings, 12,5 ml each) Per serving: 35kJ; 0,8 g carbohydrate; 0,7 g protein; 0,2 g fat; 0 mg cholesterol; 0,1 g fibre Exchanges: free

DIABETIC CUSTARD

For a thicker custard – for piping or spreading – increase custard powder to 50 ml. For a thinner, pouring custard, decrease powder to 25 ml, with the same amount of milk.

500 ml skim milk
19 g (37,5 ml) custard powder
4 ml liquid artificial sweetener *or* to taste

Using 75 ml of the milk, mix to a paste with custard powder in a large mixing-bowl. Bring remaining milk to the boil. Pour *immediately* over custard powder paste, stirring quickly. It will thicken at once. If not, return custard to saucepan, and cook over medium heat,

stirring continuously, until thickened. Sweeten to taste and serve hot.

Makes 300 ml, or 24 by 12,5 ml servings

(Based on 24 servings, 12,5 ml each) Per serving: 45kJ; 1,4 g carbohydrate; 0,8 g protein; 0,1 g fat; 0 mg cholesterol; 0,2 g fibre Exchanges: free

STRAWBERRY SAUCE

250 ml water
165 g (125 ml) diabetic strawberry jam
juice of half a lemon
10 g (20 ml) cornflour, mixed to a paste with
37,5 ml water, extra

Place water, jam and lemon juice in a small saucepan. Bring to the boil, stirring. Add cornflour paste, stir well. Return to the boil. Cook, stirring, until thickened. Serve hot, over ice-cream, canned pears or peaches.

Makes 375 ml, or 30 by 12,5 ml servings

(Based on 30 servings, 12,5 ml each) Per serving: 65kJ; 3,9 g carbohydrate; 0 g protein; 0 g fat; 0 mg cholesterol; 0,1 g fibre Exchanges: free

◄ Clockwise from back right: Chocolate sauce; Diabetic custard; Strawberry sauce

MINT SAUCE

Serve with grilled meat or roast lamb.

250 ml chopped fresh mint leaves
50 ml brown vinegar
125 ml water
12 drops liquid artificial sweetener
salt and freshly ground black pepper to taste

Place all ingredients in a small saucepan, bring to the boil. Boil gently, five minutes. Adjust seasoning to taste. Pour into a heatproof jug, leave to cool. Serve at room temperature.

Makes 250 ml, or 25 by 10 ml servings

Exchanges: free

GARLIC AND PARSLEY DRESSING

75 ml olive-oil
5 ml salt
3 ml freshly ground black pepper
6 drops liquid artificial sweetener
50 ml white wine vinegar
25 ml finely chopped parsley
2 cloves of garlic, crushed

Place all ingredients in a screw-top jar, shake well. Store, sealed, in the refrigerator.

Makes about 140 ml, or 14 by 10 ml servings

(Based on 14 servings, 10 ml each) Per serving: 185kJ;
0 g carbohydrate; 0 g protein; 5 g fat; 0 mg cholesterol
Exchanges: 1 fat

WHIPPED TOPPING

Serve with fruit or jelly.

125 ml ice-cold water
50 g (125 ml) skim milk powder
3 ml liquid artificial sweetener
5 ml lemon juice
1 ml vanilla essence

Chill mixing-bowl and beaters in freezer, 30 minutes. Place water and milk powder in chilled bowl, beat until mixture begins to thicken. Add sweetener, lemon juice and vanilla essence, beat until stiff. Use immediately.

Makes 450 ml, or 9 by 50 ml servings

(Based on nine servings, 50 ml each) Per serving: 153kJ; 5,3 g carbohydrate; 3,6 g protein; 0,1 g fat; 2 mg cholesterol; 0 g fibre
Exchanges: 1/2 skim milk

HOME-MADE TOMATO SAUCE

410 g can whole peeled tomatoes, undrained and chopped
2 onions, finely chopped
3 ml dried sweet basil
3 ml dried thyme
1 clove of garlic, crushed
salt and freshly ground black pepper to taste
8 drops liquid artificial sweetener, *or* to taste

Place all ingredients in a saucepan, bring to the boil, stirring frequently. Reduce heat, simmer, uncovered, until thick and pulpy. Purée in blender or electric food processor, if desired. Adjust seasoning and sweetener to taste. Serve hot or cold.

Makes 625 ml, or 50 by 12,5 ml servings

(Based on 50 servings, 12,5 ml each) Per serving: 15kJ;
0,7 g carbohydrate; 0,2 g protein; 0 g fat; 0 mg cholesterol; 0,2 g fibre
Exchanges: free

GREEN YOGHURT DRESSING

Use as a salad dressing, or as an accompanying sauce for chicken or fish.

150 ml low-fat plain yoghurt
juice of half a lemon
3 ml prepared English mustard
salt and freshly ground black pepper to taste
25 ml finely chopped onion
25 ml finely chopped capers
25 ml finely chopped parsley

Combine all ingredients in a screw-top jar, shake well. Purée in blender or electric food processor, if desired. Store in refrigerator.

Makes 200 ml, or 20 by 10 ml servings

Variation
For a plainer dressing, omit onion, capers and parsley.

(Based on 20 servings, 10 ml each) Per serving: 24kJ;
0,8 g carbohydrate; 0,4 g protein; 0,1 g fat; 0 mg cholesterol; 0 g fibre
Exchanges: free

CREAM SUBSTITUTE

Use as a filling, or for decorating cakes, tarts or desserts.

410 g can unsweetened evaporated milk
15 g (25 ml) gelatine, soaked in
50 ml water
liquid artificial sweetener to taste

Heat milk in a saucepan, just until a skin forms. Stir in soaked gelatine, heat until melted. Strain milk into a bowl, leave to cool. Chill over ice until beginning to thicken. Pour into mixer-bowl, whip until stiff, adding

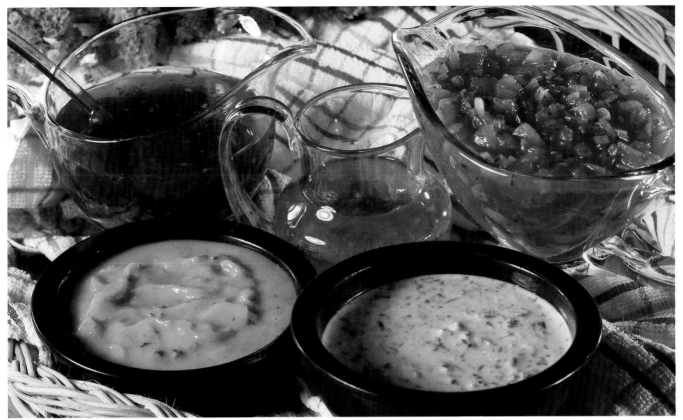

Clockwise from back left: Mint sauce; Garlic and parsley dressing; Home-made tomato sauce; Green yoghurt dressing; Curry sauce

sweetener to taste. Use immediately, or store, covered, in the refrigerator for a few days.

Makes about 375 ml

Per 375 ml: 2 214kJ; 34,4 g carbohydrate; 34,5 g protein; 27,2 g fat; 105 mg cholesterol; 0 g fibre
Exchanges: 9 whole milk

CURRY SAUCE

Serve with hard-boiled egg-halves, baked potatoes, steamed mixed vegetables, grilled meat or chicken.

10 ml sunflower oil
1 onion, finely sliced
15 g (30 ml) wholewheat flour
12,5 ml mild curry-powder
5 drops liquid artificial sweetener
2 ml salt
freshly ground black pepper to taste
3 ml ground ginger
3 ml turmeric
325 ml skim milk
10 ml freshly squeezed lemon juice
10 ml finely chopped parsley

Heat oil in a saucepan, sauté onion two minutes. Stir in next seven ingredients, cook, stirring, one minute. Remove from heat, stir in milk. Return to heat, bring to the boil, stirring continuously. Cook two minutes.

Remove from heat, stir in lemon juice and parsley, serve hot.

Makes 375 ml, or 10 by 37,5 ml servings

(Based on 10 servings, 37,5 ml each) Per serving: 147kJ; 4,1 g carbohydrate; 1,6 g protein; 1,2 g fat; 1 mg cholesterol; 0,7 g fibre
Exchanges: free

SPICY SALAD DRESSING

As a healthy and easy alternative, squeeze fresh lemon juice over a tossed green salad – makes a delicious dressing, with no other seasoning necessary.

60 ml sunflower oil
37,5 ml olive-oil
37,5 ml freshly squeezed lemon juice
25 ml brown vinegar
4-5 drops liquid artificial sweetener
3 ml dried coriander
5 ml cumin seeds
1 clove of garlic, crushed
salt and freshly ground black pepper to taste

Place all ingredients in a screw-top jar, shake well. Store, sealed, in the refrigerator.

Makes 160 ml, or 16 by 10 ml servings

(Based on 16 servings, 10 ml each) Per serving: 374kJ; 0,3 g carbohydrate; 0 g protein; 10 g fat; 0 mg cholesterol; 0 g fibre
Exchanges: 2 fat

BASIC WHITE SAUCE

15 g margarine
12 g (25 ml) wholewheat flour
300 ml skim milk
salt and pepper to taste

Step 1:

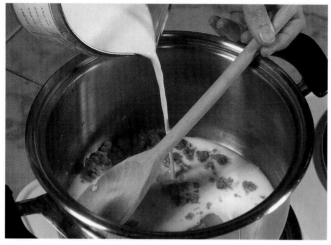

Melt margarine in a small saucepan, stir in flour, cook one minute. Add milk, stir well.

Step 2:

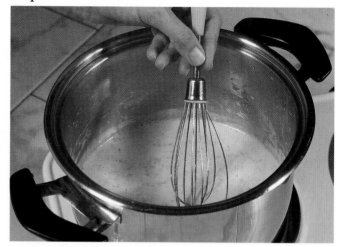

Using a wire whisk, whisk sauce over medium heat until it comes to the boil. Cook one to two minutes until thick and smooth. Season.

Variations
Caper sauce
Add 25 ml capers and 12,5 ml caper vinegar. Serve with boiled mutton or fish.

Cheese sauce
Stir in 50 g (125 ml) grated low-fat cheese. Serve on toast, or with cauliflower or fish.

Mushroom sauce
Sauté 100 g chopped mushrooms in the margarine before adding the flour. Use stock instead of milk, and serve with grilled meat or as a toast topping.

Mustard sauce
Add 10 ml prepared French mustard and 5 ml prepared English mustard when adding the flour. Good with pork or oily fish.

Parsley sauce
Stir in 25 ml finely chopped parsley. Serve with boiled mutton or fish.

Step 3:

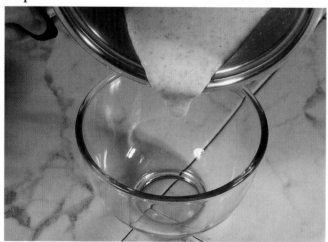

This sauce is of a good, pouring consistency. For a coating sauce, increase margarine and flour to 30 g each, and for piping or filling, increase margarine and flour to 45 g each, keeping milk quantity the same.

Makes 300 ml

Per 300 ml: 1 059kJ; 21,9 g carbohydrate; 11,8 g protein; 13 g fat;
6 mg cholesterol; 1,5 g fibre
Exchanges: 1 skim milk; 1 starch; 3 fat

DIABETIC MAYONNAISE

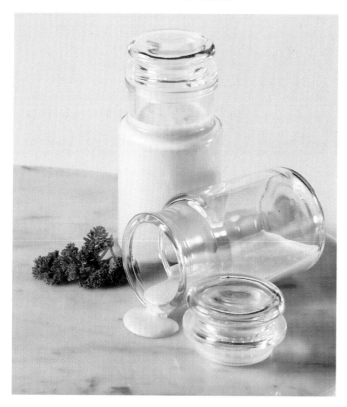

125 g low-fat smooth cottage cheese
175 ml carton low-fat plain yoghurt
12,5 ml white wine vinegar
3 ml prepared French mustard
juice of half a lemon
2 ml garlic salt
2 ml celery salt
good grinding of black pepper
4-6 drops liquid artificial sweetener *or* to taste

Place all ingredients in an electric blender or a food processor. Blend until smooth. Adjust seasoning and sweetness to taste. Pour into a clean, dry jar, refrigerate until required. Stir, shake or whisk well before using.

Makes about 250 ml, or 25 by 10 ml servings

(Based on 25 servings, 10 ml each) Per serving: 44kJ; 0,8 g carbohydrate; 1 g protein; 0,3 g fat; 1 mg cholesterol; 0 g fibre Exchanges: free

TANGY BARBECUE SAUCE

Serve with grilled meat, fish or poultry; baked potato; vegetarian dish; or savoury-filled pancake.

10 ml sunflower oil
1 onion, finely chopped
2 cloves of garlic, crushed
1 red pepper, seeded and diced
25 ml tarragon vinegar *or* red wine vinegar
25 ml Worcestershire sauce
150 ml home-made beef stock (see Pg 26)
150 ml tomato juice
10 ml prepared English mustard
salt and freshly ground black pepper to taste
pinch of chilli-powder (optional)
8 drops liquid artificial sweetener *or* to taste

Heat oil in a saucepan, sauté onion and garlic, three to four minutes. Add red pepper, fry a further two minutes, stirring. Stir in vinegar, Worcestershire sauce, stock, tomato juice, mustard and seasonings, bring to the boil. Reduce heat, cover and simmer 15 minutes. Add sweetener to taste. Serve hot or cold.

Makes about 450 ml, or 18 by 25 ml servings

(Based on 18 servings, 25 ml each) Per serving: 21kJ; 0,9 g carbohydrate; 0,2 g protein; 0 g fat; 0 mg cholesterol; 0,2 g fibre Exchanges: free

FRENCH DRESSING

50 ml sunflower oil
50 ml water
37,5 ml cider vinegar
1 clove of garlic, crushed (optional)
salt and freshly ground black pepper to taste
8 drops liquid artificial sweetener
3 ml prepared English mustard
1 ml cayenne pepper

Place all ingredients in a screw-top jar, shake well. Store, sealed, in the refrigerator.

Makes 150 ml, or 15 by 10 ml servings

(Based on 15 servings, 10 ml each) Per serving: 148kJ; 0 g carbohydrate; 0 g protein; 0,5 g fat; 0 mg cholesterol; 0 g fibre Exchanges: 1/2 fat

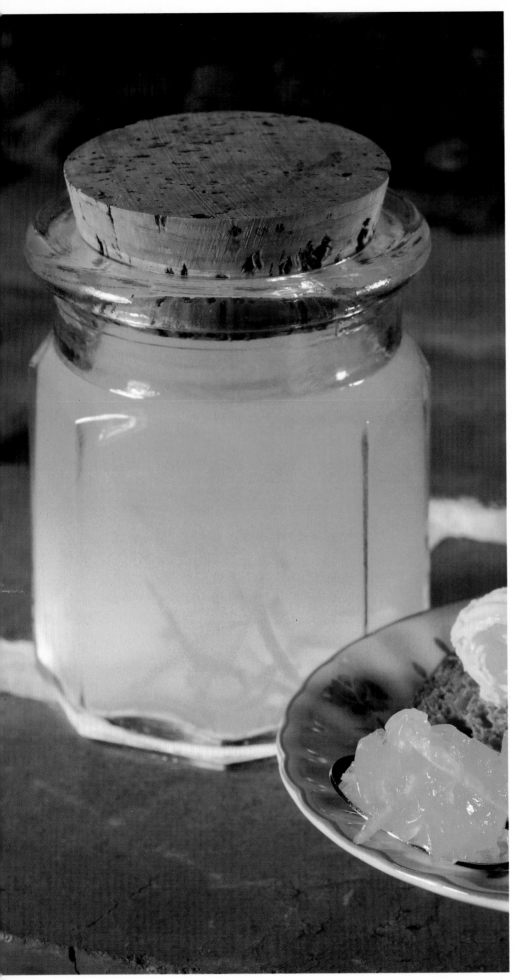

ORANGE AND LEMON MARMALADE

This version makes a clearer, less chunky marmalade. Finely shredded rind is suspended in orange jelly, the remaining fruit being discarded before bottling.

4 small oranges
2 large lemons
1 litre water
15 g (25 ml) gelatine, soaked in
75 ml water, extra
25 ml liquid artificial
    sweetener *or* to taste

Thinly peel oranges and lemons, cut rind into fine shreds. Cook rind in 400 ml water, covered, 20 minutes. Set aside.
Chop rest of fruit roughly, place in a large saucepan with 600 ml water. Bring to the boil, press down firmly with potato masher. Reduce heat, cover and simmer 40 minutes. Leave to cool completely. Empty into a well-padded jelly-bag, allow to drip through slowly overnight – do not disturb.
Strain collected liquid through double layer of muslin into saucepan, add reserved rind. Discard fruit remaining in bag.
Stir soaked gelatine and sweetener into rind mixture, cook five minutes, until mixture is boiling and gelatine has dissolved. Remove from heat, allow to cool. Chill until just beginning to thicken. Spoon into hot, dry, sterilised jars, making sure shredded rind is evenly distributed throughout jelly. Leave until cold and set. Cover surface with a round of wax-paper dipped in brandy, seal and label. Store in refrigerator.

Makes about 750 ml, or 75 by 10 ml servings

(Based on 75 servings, 10 ml each)
Per serving: 18kJ; 1 g carbohydrate; 0,2 g protein; 0 g fat; 0 mg cholesterol; 0,1 g fibre
Exchanges: free

PRESERVES

Included are jams, chutneys, pickles and relishes, designed to add zest and flavour to your meals. Used sparingly, the additional kilojoules are negligible, and need not be added to your daily total.
These sugar-free preserves do not have the keeping quality of the sugar-loaded ones, and must be stored in the refrigerator, where they will keep for several days.

ONION RELISH

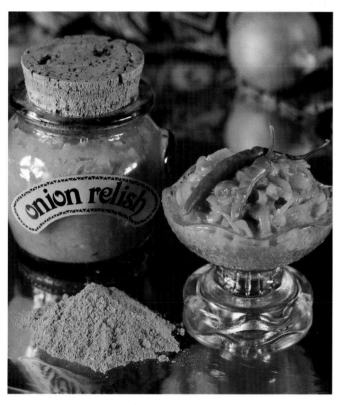

750 g onions, thinly sliced
20 g margarine
40 g fresh ginger, peeled and finely chopped
15 ml hot curry-powder *or* **to taste**
5 ml liquid artificial sweetener *or* **to taste**
250 ml dry white wine *or* **white wine vinegar**
75 ml white wine vinegar
salt to taste
1 green *or* **red chilli, seeded and chopped**

Sauté onions in melted margarine until softened, but not brown. Stir in ginger and curry-powder, cook one minute, stirring. Add remaining ingredients, bring to the boil. Reduce heat and simmer, uncovered, 20 to 30 minutes, or until thick, stirring frequently. Remove from heat, adjust seasoning to taste, spoon into a hot, dry, sterilised jar. Remove any air bubbles, seal at once. Allow to cool, label and store in refrigerator.

Makes about 500 ml, or 50 by 10 ml servings

(Based on 50 servings, 10 ml each) Per serving: 45kJ; 1,5 g carbohydrate; 0,2 g protein; 0 g fat; 0 mg cholesterol; 0,2 g fibre
Exchanges: free

STRAWBERRY JAM

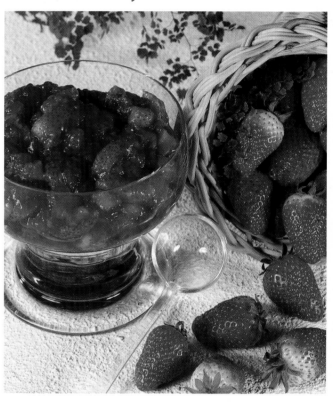

Use other fresh berries instead of strawberries, if preferred. Store jam in refrigerator for up to two weeks. Use within a week of opening.
500 g fresh strawberries, washed, hulled and roughly chopped
12,5 ml fresh lemon juice
6 g (10 ml) gelatine, soaked in
30 ml water
8 ml liquid artificial sweetener *or* **to taste**
3 ml vanilla essence

Place strawberries and lemon juice in a saucepan, cook gently three minutes. Stir in soaked gelatine, stir until dissolved. Add sweetener to taste, remove from heat. Stir in vanilla essence, pour into a hot, dry, sterilised jar, allow to cool slightly. Cover with a round of wax-paper dipped in brandy, leave to cool completely. Seal, label and store in refrigerator.

Makes about 400 ml, or 40 by 10 ml servings

(Based on 40 servings, 10 ml each) Per serving: 10kJ; 0,4 g carbohydrate; 0 g protein; 0 g fat; 0 mg cholesterol; 0,2 g fibre
Exchanges: free

RHUBARB AND APPLE JAM

Use 10 ml per serving.

250 g fresh rhubarb, trimmed and roughly chopped
500 g cooking apples
500 ml water
20 ml liquid artificial sweetener *or* to taste
6 g (10 ml) gelatine, soaked in
30 ml water, extra

Place rhubarb in a saucepan. Peel, core and dice apples, reserve skins and cores. Add diced apple to rhubarb, pour in water. Bring to the boil. Reduce heat, simmer, uncovered, 40 minutes, stirring occasionally. Meanwhile, place apple skins and cores in a small saucepan, cover with water. Simmer gently, 15 minutes, strain.
Add strained liquid to rhubarb mixture. Stir in soaked gelatine, stir over heat until dissolved. Remove from heat, pour into a hot, dry, sterilised jar. Allow to cool three minutes, cover surface with a round of wax-paper dipped in brandy. Leave to cool completely. Seal, label and store in refrigerator.

Makes 500 ml, or 50 by 10 ml servings

(Based on 50 servings, 10 ml each) Per serving: 25kJ; 1,3 g carbohydrate; 0 g protein; 0 g fat; 0 mg cholesterol; 0,3 g fibre Exchanges: free

APRICOT AND PINEAPPLE JAM

250 g dried apricots
600 ml water
500 ml freshly cubed pineapple, hard core discarded
30 g (50 ml) blanched almonds, roughly chopped
juice of one large lemon
25 ml liquid artificial sweetener *or* to taste

Soak apricots in water overnight. Place apricots with water in a large saucepan, add pineapple. Bring to the boil. Reduce heat, simmer, uncovered, about 25 minutes, until thick. Transfer to bowl of food processor, blend for a few seconds, just until coarsely chopped. Return mixture to saucepan, add almonds and lemon juice, simmer three minutes. Add sweetener, stir well. Remove from heat, cool slightly. Pour into a hot, dry, sterilised jar, cover surface with a round of wax-paper dipped in brandy. Seal when cold, label and store in refrigerator.

Makes about 650 ml, or 65 by 10 ml servings

(Based on 65 servings, 10 ml each) Per serving: 59kJ; 3,2 g carbohydrate; 0,1 g protein; 0 g fat; 0 mg cholesterol; 0,4 g fibre Exchanges: free

PEAR AND ORANGE JAM

Store in refrigerator for up to two weeks. Use within a week of opening.

750 ml unsweetened pear juice
1 box diabetic jelly powder (orange flavour)
  sufficient to set about one litre of liquid
  (see instructions on box)
5 ml liquid artificial sweetener *or* to taste
12,5 ml finely chopped fresh mint
10 ml finely grated orange rind

Bring pear juice to the boil. Stir in jelly powder, stir until dissolved. Add sweetener, mint and orange rind, stir well. Remove from heat, cool slightly. Pour into a hot, dry, sterilised jar, cover surface of jam with a round of wax-paper dipped in brandy. Leave to cool completely. Seal, label and store in refrigerator.

Makes 750 ml, or 75 by 10 ml servings

(Based on 75 servings, 10 ml each) Per serving: 20kJ; 1,2 g carbohydrate; 0 g protein; 0 g fat; 0 mg cholesterol; 0 g fibre Exchanges: free

THREE-FRUIT MARMALADE

2 large oranges
1 large lemon
1 large grapefruit
750 ml water
15 g (25 ml) gelatine, soaked in
75 ml water, extra
25 ml liquid artificial sweetener *or* to taste

Thinly peel oranges, lemon and grapefruit. Slice rind into very fine shreds, enough to make 250 ml, place remainder in a muslin bag. Cut away all pith from fruit, add to muslin bag. Chop fruit finely, add pips to muslin bag, tie securely with string. Place shredded rind, chopped fruit, muslin bag and water, in a large, glass bowl, cover, leave overnight.

Turn contents of bowl into a large saucepan, cook, stirring, until rind is soft, about 15 minutes. Squeeze liquid from muslin bag, remove and discard. Stir in soaked gelatine, cook a further five minutes, stirring. Add sweetener, remove from heat. Allow to cool slightly, pour into hot, dry, sterilised jars. Allow to cool five minutes. Cover surface of jam with a round of wax-paper dipped in brandy, leave to cool completely. Seal, label and store in refrigerator.

Makes about 1,25 litres, or 125 by 10 ml servings

(Based on 125 servings, 10 ml each) Per serving: 11kJ; 0,6 g carbohydrate; 0 g protein; 0 g fat; 0 mg cholesterol; 0,1 g fibre Exchanges: free

Clockwise from back left: Rhubarb and apple jam; Pear and orange jam; Three-fruit marmalade; Apricot and pineapple jam ▶

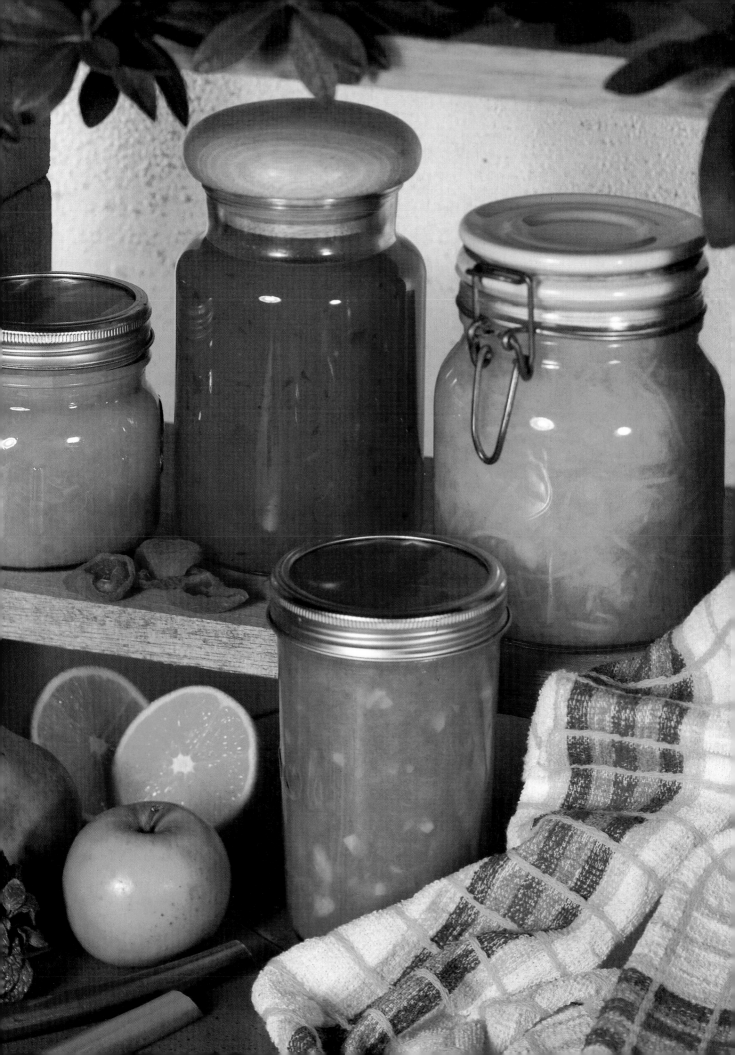

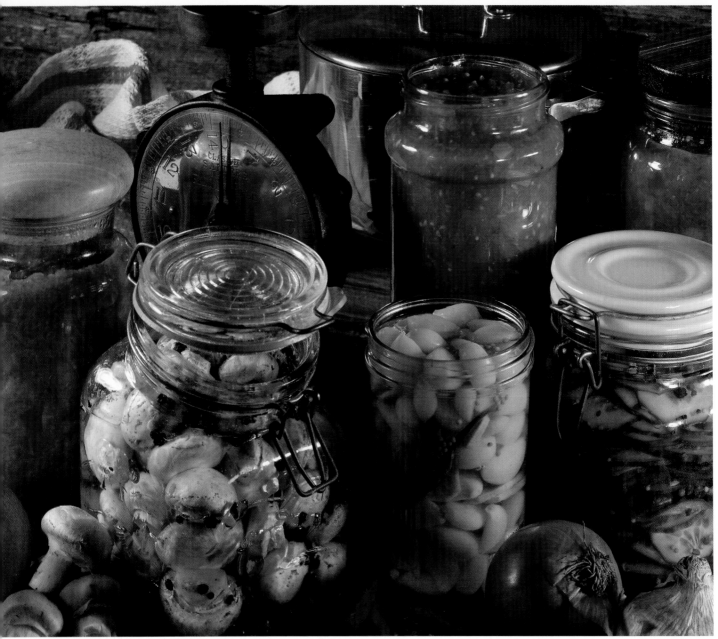

Clockwise from back left: Hot orange chutney; Green tomato chutney; Uncooked spicy cucumber pickles; Pickled garlic; Pickled Mushroom

PICKLED GARLIC

A wonderful way to preserve garlic – it looks attractive on the shelf, too. Bottle in small quantities to ensure you have a constant supply. Will keep indefinitely if bottled correctly; but, once opened, must be stored in refrigerator and used within three to four weeks.

800 g garlic heads, separated into cloves, unpeeled
85 g fresh ginger, peeled and thinly sliced
200 ml coarse salt
4 chillies
250 ml white wine vinegar
125 ml dry white wine *or* vinegar
12,5 ml mustard seeds

Place garlic cloves in a large saucepan with enough water to cover. Bring to the boil, boil two minutes. Drain and peel cloves. Place in a non-metallic bowl, add ginger and salt, mix well. Cover and refrigerate 48 hours. Drain, rinse well under cold running water, pat dry. Pack ginger and garlic into clean, dry, sterilised jars, adding one or two chillies to each jar.
Combine remaining ingredients in a saucepan, bring to the boil. Fill jars to overflowing with hot mixture, remove air bubbles. Seal immediately, and leave to cool completely. Label and store in a cool, dark place until required.

Makes 750 ml

Per clove of garlic: 6kJ; 0,3 g carbohydrate; 0,1 g protein; 0 g fat; 0 mg cholesterol; 0 g fibre
Exchanges: free

98

UNCOOKED SPICY CUCUMBER PICKLES

Will keep for up to one week in refrigerator.

3 small cucumbers, thinly sliced
salt
250 ml boiling water
30 ml mixed pickling spices
1 onion, thinly sliced
1 clove of garlic, crushed
340 ml dry apple cider
45 ml cider vinegar
5 ml liquid artificial sweetener *or* to taste

Place cucumber slices in a large glass bowl. Sprinkle with salt, toss well. Cover, set aside 30 minutes. Rinse well under cold, running water, pat dry.
Pour boiling water over pickling spices, set aside 30 minutes.
Combine all ingredients, stir gently to blend. Pack into a hot, dry, sterilised jar, seal. Label and store in refrigerator for at least 24 hours before using.

Makes 750 ml, or 15 by 50 ml servings

(Based on 15 servings, 50 ml each) Per serving: 74kJ; 2,4 g carbohydrate; 0,3 g protein; 0 g fat; 0 mg cholesterol; 0,5 g fibre
Exchanges: free

HOT ORANGE CHUTNEY

7 large navel oranges
1 large lemon
5 Granny Smith apples
3 onions, chopped
1 litre brown vinegar
35 ml liquid artificial sweetener *or* to taste
250 g (415 ml) sultanas
75 ml grated fresh ginger
6 cloves of garlic, crushed
2 red peppers, seeded and diced *or* canned pimientos, chopped
25 ml turmeric
7 ml freshly ground black pepper
5 ml cayenne pepper
5 ml salt

Grate zest off oranges and lemon, remove and discard all pith. Chop fruit finely, discard pips. Peel, core and chop apples. Place grated zest and chopped fruit in a large saucepan. Add remaining ingredients, bring to the boil. Reduce heat, simmer gently about one hour, stirring occasionally, until thick. Ladle into hot, dry, sterilised jars. Remove air bubbles, seal immediately. Allow to cool, label and store in refrigerator.

Makes 1,5 litres, or 150 by 10 ml servings

(Based on 150 servings, 10 ml each) Per serving: 60kJ; 3,2 g carbohydrate; 0,2 g protein; 0 g fat; 0 mg cholesterol; 0,4 g fibre
Exchanges: free

GREEN TOMATO CHUTNEY

2 kg green tomatoes, chopped
500 ml cider vinegar
10 ml salt
2 large onions, chopped
12,5 ml hot curry-powder *or* to taste
10 ml whole allspice
10 ml mustard seeds
5 ml ground ginger
freshly ground black pepper to taste
10 ml liquid artificial sweetener *or* to taste
2 green *or* red chillies, whole

Place all ingredients, except the last two, in a large saucepan. Cook over low heat, stirring well. Bring to the boil. Reduce heat, simmer steadily about one hour, or until thick. Remove from heat, add sweetener to taste. Ladle into hot, dry, sterilised jars, push a chilli down side of each jar. Remove air bubbles, seal at once. Allow to cool, label and store in refrigerator.

Makes 1,5 litres, or 150 by 10 ml servings

(Based on 150 servings, 10 ml each) Per serving: 18kJ; 0,7 g carbohydrate; 0,1 g protein; 0 g fat; 0 mg cholesterol; 0,2 g fibre
Exchanges: free

PICKLED MUSHROOMS

May be stored on the pantry shelf for up to six months, if bottled correctly. Keep in refrigerator once opened, and use within a week.

400 g button mushrooms, wiped and stalks trimmed
salt water
750 ml white vinegar
15 g (25 ml) black peppercorns
1 ml cayenne pepper
30 g fresh ginger, peeled and grated

Rinse mushrooms in lightly salted water, drain well. Boil vinegar, peppercorns, cayenne pepper and ginger, five minutes. Add mushrooms, simmer gently five minutes. Pack mushrooms into hot, dry, sterilised jars, pour over boiling liquid until it overflows. Remove air bubbles, seal at once. Leave to cool completely. Label and store in a cool, dark place until required.

Makes one litre

Per button mushroom: 7kJ; 0,3 g carbohydrate; 0,1 g protein; 0 g fat; 0 mg cholesterol; 0,1 g fibre
Exchanges: free

SEE PAGE 110 FOR MAKING JAM IN SMALL QUANTITIES.

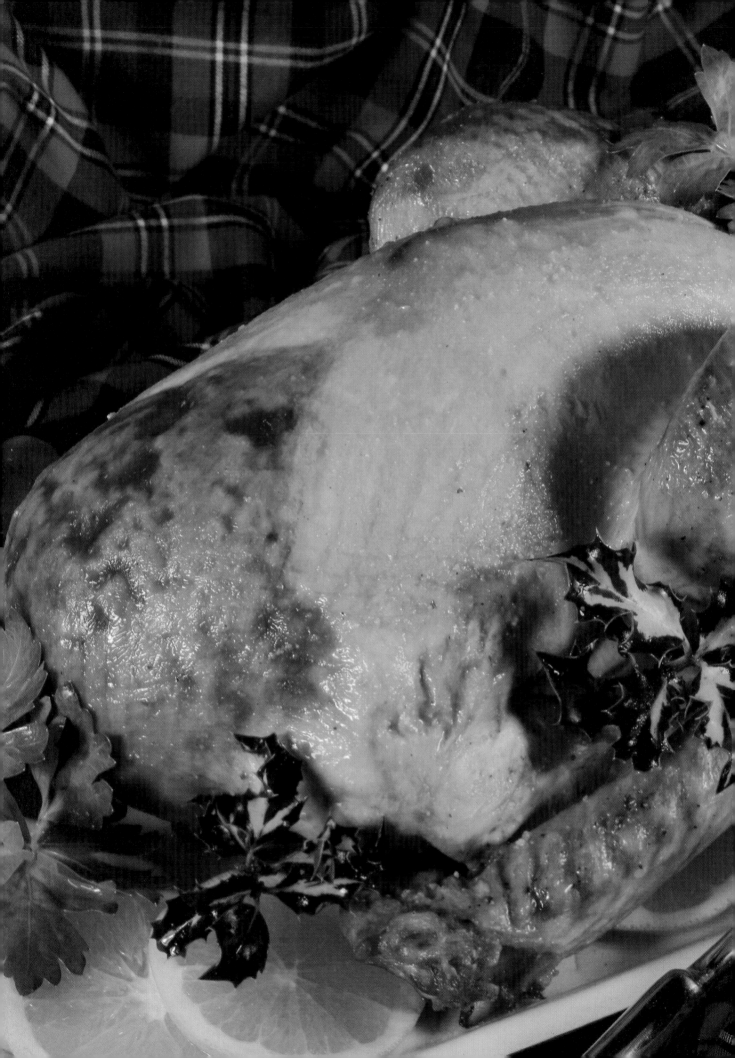

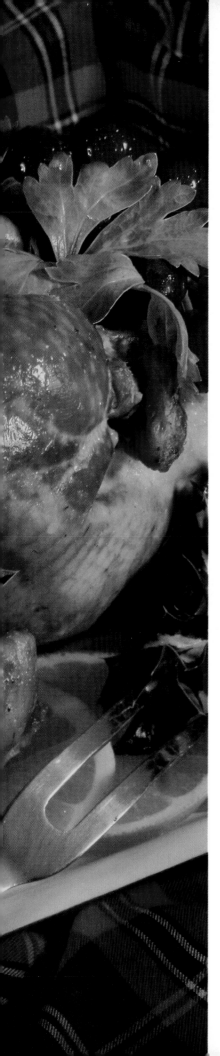

SPECIAL OCCASIONS

Everyone likes to celebrate heydays and holidays – diabetics are no exception. Here are ideas for Christmas, Easter and Valentine's Day the whole family can enjoy.
While far healthier than the conventional, mega-kilojoule bakes for such events, many of these are high in fat, and should be viewed for what they are: special-occasion fare.

ROAST TURKEY

Remember to remove skin before serving.

4 kg turkey, washed and dried
salt and freshly ground black pepper

Chestnut stuffing
285 g can unsweetened chestnuts, roughly chopped
250 g beef sausages, skinned
30 g slice wholewheat bread, crumbed
salt and pepper

Celery and walnut stuffing
6 x 30 g wholewheat bread slices, crumbed
50 g (125 ml) walnuts, roughly chopped
4 celery stalks, finely chopped
5 ml dried tarragon
5 ml finely grated orange rind
50 ml fresh orange juice
salt and pepper

To complete
30 g margarine
500 ml home-made chicken stock (see Pg 34) *or* water
500 ml dry white wine *or* dry apple cider

Season turkey inside and out, set aside. Combine all ingredients for Chestnut Stuffing, stuff crop end of turkey. Combine all ingredients for Celery and Walnut Stuffing, stuff body cavity. Truss turkey, place in a lightly greased roasting-pan.
Combine margarine, stock and wine in a saucepan, bring to the boil. Pour over turkey in pan, cover with foil, shiny side inside. Roast at 200 °C, on lowest shelf of oven, 30 minutes. Reduce temperature to 180 °C, roast about two-and-three-quarter hours, or 40 minutes per kilogram. Baste well every hour.
Remove turkey to warmed serving platter, keep warm.
Boil remaining liquid in roasting-pan over high heat until reduced by half. Adjust seasoning to taste, pour into gravy-boat, serve separately.

Serves 10

Per serving of turkey with Chestnut Stuffing: 2 667kJ; 22,8 g carbohydrate; 64,8 g protein; 29,5 g fat; 187 mg cholesterol; 3,2 g fibre
Exchanges: 30 g turkey per 1 meat exchange; 1/2 meat; 1 fat
Per serving of turkey with Celery and Walnut Stuffing: 1 847kJ; 9,4 g carbohydrate; 64,5 g protein; 14,7 g fat; 161 mg cholesterol; 1,6 g fibre
Exchanges: 30 g turkey per 1 meat exchange; 1/2 bread; 1/2 fat

WHOLEWHEAT FLAKY PASTRY

100 g (200 ml) wholewheat flour, sifted and husks
  replaced
80 g (160 ml) flour, sifted
pinch of salt
80 g margarine
squeeze of lemon juice
iced water to mix

Step 1:

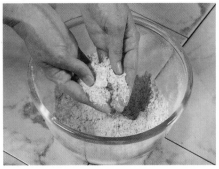

Sift together flours and salt into a mixing-bowl. Rub in
30 g margarine.

Step 2:

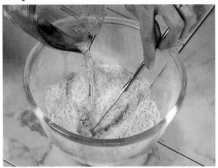

Add lemon juice to iced water. Add enough of the water
to the flour mixture to make a firm, pliable dough,
mixing with a round-bladed knife.

Step 3:

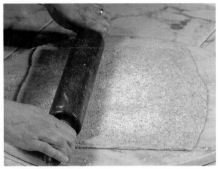

Turn out dough on to a lightly floured surface, roll out
thinly into a rectangle.

Step 4:

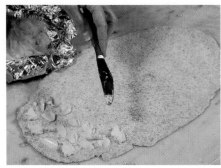

Divide remaining margarine in half. Mark dough into
three equal sections, dot one portion of margarine over
two-thirds, leaving one-third plain.

Step 5:

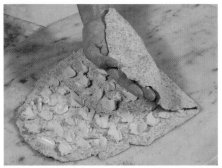

Starting with plain end, fold one-third of the dough over
the centre third. Repeat with other side.

Step 6:

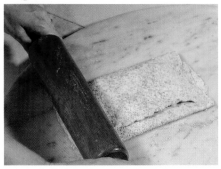

Give pastry half a turn, so that one open end is towards
you. Roll out again, and again fold into three, this time
without margarine. Wrap in clingwrap, chill 30 minutes
in refrigerator.

To complete
Repeat rolling and folding procedure, using remaining
margarine. Roll and fold again without margarine, wrap
and chill 30 minutes. Pastry is now ready to use.

Per recipe: 5 047kJ; 121,1 g carbohydrate; 20,5 g protein; 67,6 g fat;
0 mg cholesterol; 14,8 g fibre
Exchanges: 9 starch; 16 fat

CHRISTMAS PUDDING

Make at least three weeks beforehand, to allow flavours to mature.

80 g (135 ml) currants
80 g (135 ml) raisins
80 g (135 ml) sultanas
125 g (250 ml) wholewheat flour, sifted and husks replaced
120 g (500 ml) wholewheat breadcrumbs
30 g (50 ml) blanched almonds, finely chopped
5 ml ground mixed spice
5 ml ground cinnamon
3 ml ground nutmeg
3 ml bicarbonate of soda
1 large carrot, scraped and grated
finely grated rind and juice of one lemon
90 g margarine, melted
2 extra-large eggs, beaten
150 ml Guinness Stout
3 ml liquid artificial sweetener *or* to taste

Combine first 10 ingredients in a large mixing-bowl. Stir in grated carrot. Combine remaining ingredients in a small bowl, beat well. Pour into fruit mixture, stir well.
Turn mixture into a lightly greased 600 ml pudding basin. Cover with a round of pleated greaseproof paper, then foil, tie securely with string. Stand on a trivet or folded tea-towel in a large saucepan. Pour in enough boiling water to reach about two-thirds of the way up side of basin. Cover tightly with lid, steam for three hours, replenishing with boiling water as required.
Remove from water, leave to cool. Remove foil and paper, replace with new paper and foil, tie securely with string. Store in refrigerator or freezer until required. Steam again for one hour before serving. Serve hot, with Diabetic Custard (see Pg 89).

Serves eight

Per serving: 1 392kJ; 45,4 g carbohydrate; 7,5 g protein; 13 g fat; 59 mg cholesterol; 4,9 g fibre
Exchanges: 1 1/2 fruit; 1 starch; 2 1/2 fat

CHRISTMAS FRUIT-CAKE

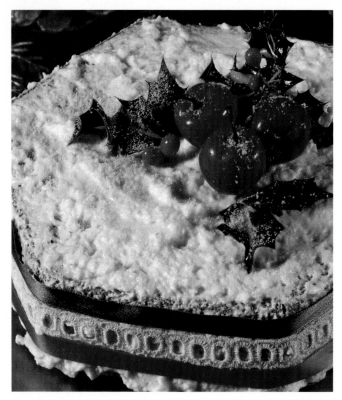

Will keep for up to three weeks, well wrapped in clingwrap and foil, and stored in an airtight tin. Cake, without marzipan or icing, may be frozen for up to six months. Quantities may be safely doubled, if desired. Substitute bran-rich self-raising flour with 125 g (250 ml) self-raising flour, 125 g (250 ml) wholewheat flour, and 8 ml baking-powder, if preferred. Hazel-nuts replace the commonly used almonds in the marzipan, as they contain less fat. Cover cake with marzipan one day before serving. Don't freeze marzipan.
The icing has a gelatine base and should be prepared on the day it is served. The Creamy Frosting on Pg 84 may be used instead.

Fruit-cake batter
250 g (500 ml) bran-rich self-raising flour, sifted
8 ml ground mixed spice
5 ml ground cinnamon
2 ml salt
50 g margarine
2 eggs
1 egg-white
5 ml liquid artificial sweetener *or* to taste
125 ml Guinness Stout
37,5 ml brandy
75 g (125 ml) sultanas
75 g (125 ml) currants
75 g (125 ml) raisins
50 g (125 ml) hazel-nuts, roughly chopped
finely grated rind of one orange
125 g carrots, scraped and finely grated

Diabetic marzipan
150 g (375 ml) hazel-nuts, ground
5 ml liquid artificial sweetener *or* to taste

30 g (60 ml) cornflour, sifted
1 extra-large egg, beaten
2 ml almond essence
25 ml diabetic apricot jam (spread), warmed and sieved

Icing
5 ml liquid artificial sweetener *or* to taste
pinch of salt
1 extra-large egg-white
3 ml freshly squeezed lemon juice
5 ml gelatine, soaked in
15 ml water

Per slice: 863kJ; 22,1 g carbohydrate· 5 g protein; 10,5 g fat; 46 mg cholesterol; 2,1 g fibre
Exchanges: 1/2 starch; 1 1/2 fat

Step 1:

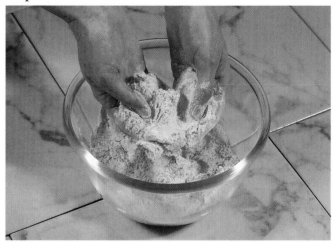

Fruit-cake batter: sift together flour, spices and salt in a mixing-bowl. Rub in margarine.

Step 2:

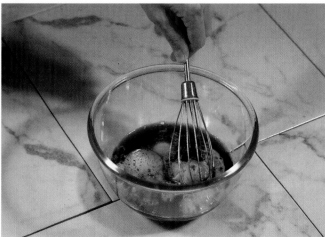

Whisk together eggs, egg-white, sweetener, stout and 25 ml of the brandy.

Step 3:

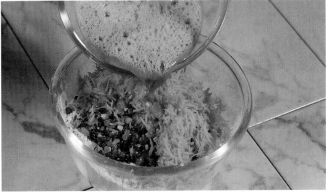

Place fruit and nuts in an electric blender or a food processor, chop roughly. Add to flour mixture with orange rind and grated carrots. Pour in egg mixture, mix well to form a soft dough.

Step 4:

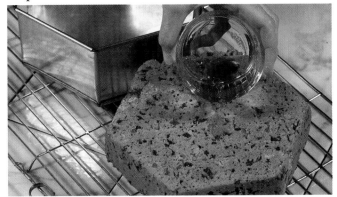

Spoon mixture into a deep, greased and base-lined 180 mm-square, round or hexagonal cake pan. Bake at 180 °C, one hour, or until a skewer inserted into the centre comes out clean. Leave to cool in pan.
Turn out on to a wire cooling rack, pierce cake all over with a skewer. Pour remaining 12,5 ml brandy over cake surface. Wrap in foil, overwrap in clingwrap. Store in airtight tin or freeze, until required.

Step 5:

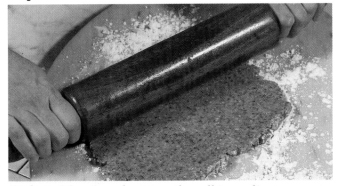

Diabetic Marzipan: beat together all ingredients except jam, work into a paste with hands. (Works well in food processor.) Roll out on a work surface dusted with cornflour.

Step 6:

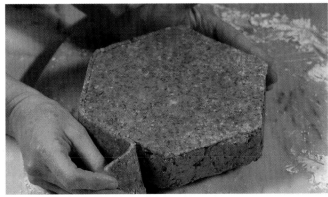

Cut to fit base and sides of cake. Cut top of cake level, invert so that base is now the top. Brush with jam, cover with marzipan. Leave for up to 12 hours before icing.

Step 7:

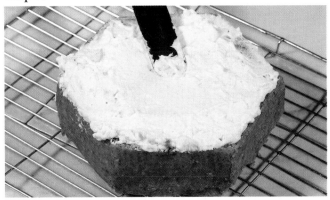

Icing: place sweetener, salt, egg-white and lemon juice in mixer-bowl. Dissolve soaked gelatine over a saucepan of simmering water, or in the microwave oven. Add to egg-white mixture. Whisk until stiff, eight to 10 minutes. Working quickly, spread icing over cake with a warmed palette knife, to give a rough finish.

To complete
Decorate top of cake with small, inedible Christmas decorations, wrap ribbon around sides. Dust with granular artificial sweetener to resemble snow, if desired. Serve at once.

Makes 20 slices

Note:
The same recipe may be used to make an Easter Simnel Cake. Use the marzipan to cover the top of the cake and roll remainder into 11 small balls, representing 11 of Jesus' apostles – Judas, who betrayed Him, is omitted.

CHRISTMAS MINCE PIES

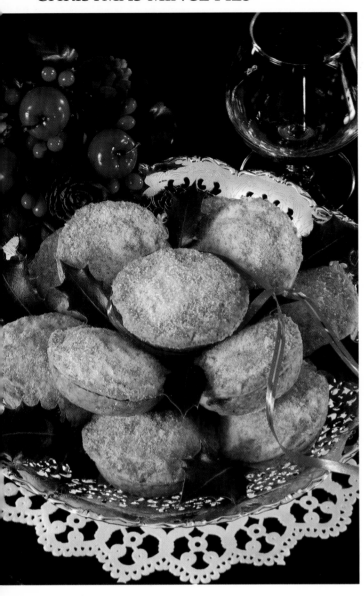

May be made using the Wholewheat Pastry on Pg 62, if preferred.

one quantity Wholewheat Flaky Pastry (see Pg 102)
one quantity Citrus Christmas Mincemeat (see Pg 107)
granular artificial sweetener to sprinkle

Per pie: 1 304kJ; 52,7 g carbohydrate; 4,7 g protein; 8,3 g fat;
0 mg cholesterol; 6,16 g fibre
Exchanges: 1 starch; 1 1/2 fat

Step 1:

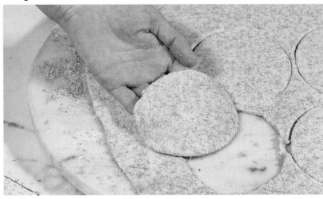

Roll out pastry thinly, cut out 12 mm by 80 mm-diameter rounds, use to line lightly greased patty-pans.

Step 2:

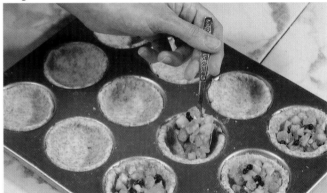

Spoon about 12,5 ml mincemeat into each.

Step 3:

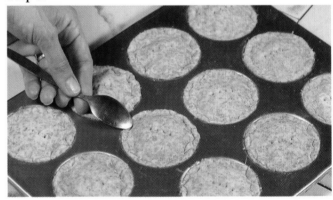

Cut out 12 mm by 75 mm-diameter rounds from remaining pastry. Dampen edges with a little water, place over mincemeat filling, seal and decorate edges with fingers or mark a pattern using a teaspoon. Prick each with a fork.

To complete
Bake at 200 °C, 25 to 30 minutes. Remove from oven, allow to cool on wire cooling racks. Sprinkle with a little granular sweetener before serving.

Makes 12

CITRUS CHRISTMAS MINCEMEAT

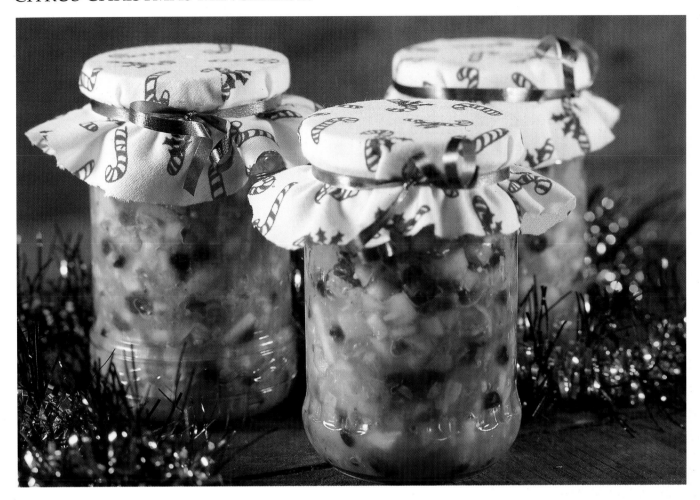

3 large lemons
2 oranges
250 g (415 ml) sultanas
90 g (150 ml) stoned dates
90 g (150 ml) raisins
90 g (150 ml) currants
3 Golden Delicious apples, peeled, cored and
　finely chopped
2 large carrots, scraped and grated
50 g (85 ml) nibbed almonds
10 ml ground mixed spice
10 ml liquid artificial sweetener *or* to taste
50 ml brandy

Peel zest off lemons and oranges, place in a small saucepan with water to cover. Bring to the boil, simmer five minutes. Drain off water, cover with fresh water, simmer a further five minutes, drain and leave to cool. This will remove any bitterness. Chop rind finely, and set aside.

Squeeze juice from lemons and oranges, set aside. Combine rind, juice and remaining ingredients, except brandy, in a mixing-bowl, stir well. Add 25 ml brandy. Adjust sweetener to taste, spoon into dry, sterilised jars. Trickle remaining brandy over surface of each jar, cover with a round of wax-paper dipped in brandy. Seal, label and store in a cool, dark place, for up to two weeks, in the refrigerator for up to four weeks, or freeze for up to one year.

Makes 500 g, or four by 500 ml jars

Per 500 ml jar: 2 694kJ; 129,4 g carbohydrate; 9,3 g protein; 8,2 g fat; 0 mg cholesterol; 14,8 g fibre
Exchanges: 8 fruit; 1 fat

WHOLEWHEAT SHORTBREAD

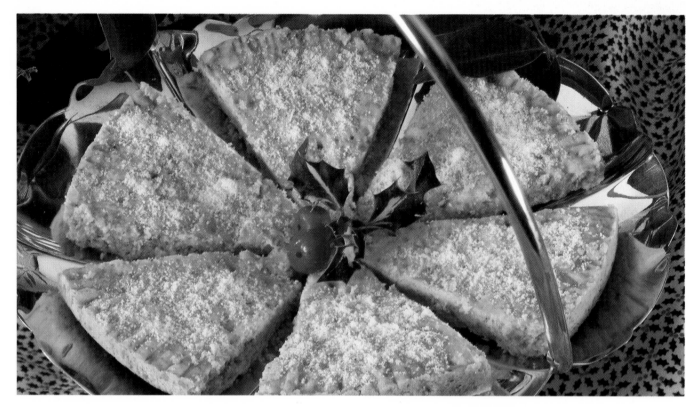

Not to be eaten by anyone on a weight-reducing diet, owing to the high fat content.

125 g (250 ml) wholewheat flour, sifted and husks
  replaced
125 g (250 ml) flour, sifted
125 g (250 ml) rice flour
250 g margarine
8 ml liquid artificial sweetener *or* to taste
granular artificial sweetener to sprinkle

Sift together flours three times. Make a mound on a clean work surface, make a well in centre. Rub in margarine until a putty-like dough is formed. Add sweetener. Divide in half. Press each half into a lightly greased 200 mm-diameter loose-bottomed cake pan. Pinch all around edges with thumb and index finger, giving a ridged border. Prick all over with a fork. Chill in refrigerator, 15 minutes.
Mark lightly into wedges with a sharp knife. Bake at 190 °C, 25 minutes. Reduce temperature to 160 °C, bake a further 20 to 25 minutes. Remove from oven, cut into wedges while hot. Leave to cool completely in pans. Sprinkle with granular artificial sweetener, remove carefully from pans. Store in airtight tins.

Makes two by 200 mm rounds, or 24 wedges

Per wedge: 525kJ; 10,7 g carbohydrate; 1,4 g protein; 8,3 g fat;
0 mg cholesterol; 0,8 g fibre
Exchanges: 1 starch; 2 fat

HOT CROSS BUNS

25 g cube fresh yeast *or* 15 ml dried yeast
350 ml lukewarm water
250 g (500 ml) flour, sifted
250 g (500 ml) wholewheat flour, sifted and husks
  replaced
3 ml salt
5 ml ground mixed spice
5 ml ground cinnamon
pinch of ground cloves
5 ml finely grated lemon rind
5 ml finely grated orange rind
60 g margarine
8 ml liquid artificial sweetener *or* to taste
1 egg, beaten
25 ml skim milk
90 g (150 ml) currants
unsweetened shortcrust pastry for crosses
25 ml skim milk for brushing

Combine yeast and lukewarm water, leave to froth in a warm, draught-free place, 15 minutes.
Sift together flours, salt and spices, add rinds. Rub in margarine. Beat together sweetener, yeast mixture, egg and milk, stir into flour mixture to make a firm dough. Turn out on to a lightly floured surface, knead five minutes. Knead in currants.
Place in a lightly oiled bowl, cover with clingwrap and a dampened tea-towel, leave in a warm, draught-free place until doubled in bulk, about one hour.
Divide into 12 equal pieces, form into balls. Arrange on a lightly greased baking tray. Cut a cross on top of each with a sharp knife. Cut thin strips of pastry, brush with

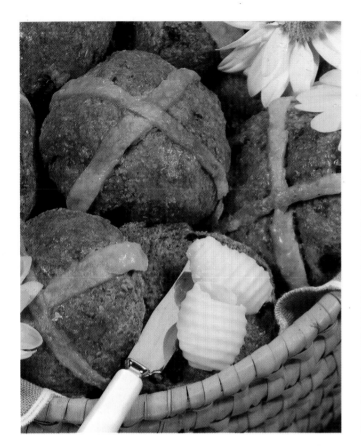

VALENTINE BISCUITS

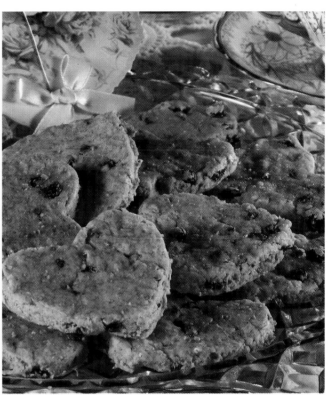

water, place in position over cut crosses. Cover, leave to rise until doubled in bulk, about 30 minutes. Bake at 220 °C, about 25 minutes, until they are well risen and sound hollow when rapped underneath with the knuckles. Brush with milk as soon as they come out of the oven. Allow to cool on a wire cooling rack, before serving, split and spread with margarine. Best eaten the same day.

Makes 12

125 g margarine
8 ml liquid artificial sweetener *or* to taste
1 egg, separated
100 g (200 ml) wholewheat flour, sifted and husks
  replaced
25 g (50 ml) flour, sifted
50 g (100 ml) rice flour
3 ml baking-powder
2 ml ground mixed spice
3 ml ground cinnamon
60 g (100 ml) currants
3 ml vanilla essence
about 20 ml skim milk

Cream together margarine, sweetener and egg-yolk. Sift together dry ingredients, beat into margarine mixture. Add currants, vanilla essence and enough milk to form a soft dough.
Knead lightly, roll out on a lightly floured surface to 6 mm thickness. Cut out heart shapes using a biscuit cutter, arrange on a lightly greased baking tray. Brush biscuits with lightly frothed egg-white, bake at 200 °C, 12 to 15 minutes. Remove to a wire cooling rack, allow to cool completely. Store in an airtight tin.

Makes 24

Variation
Make a small hole with a skewer at top end of each heart before baking. Thread small piece of ribbon through hole, tie in a small bow.

Per bun: 913kJ; 34,2 g carbohydrate; 6,4 g protein; 5,2 g fat;
21 mg cholesterol; 4,1 g fibre
Exchanges: 2 starch; 1 fat

Per biscuit: 291kJ; 6,1 g carbohydrate; 1,1 g protein; 4,4 g fat;
8 mg cholesterol; 0,6 g fibre
Exchanges: 1/2 starch; 1 fat

METRICATION CHART

Throughout this book, the following metrication measures have been used. Make use of a gram scale, or a set of metric measuring cups and spoons for best results.

Note: These conversions are approximate measures only.

WEIGHTS (MASS)

$^1/_2$ oz		15 g
1 oz		30 g
2 oz		60 g
3 oz		90 g
4 oz		125 g
5 oz		150 g
6 oz		180 g
7 oz		210 g
8 oz	half a pound (lb)	
8 oz		250 g
1 lb		500 g
2 lb		1 kg
1 000g		1 kg

VOLUME

$^1/_8$	cup	30 ml
$^1/_4$	cup	60 ml
$^1/_3$	cup	80 ml
$^1/_2$	cup	125 ml
$^2/_3$	cup	170 ml
$^3/_4$	cup	190 ml
1	cup	250 ml
1	cup	8 fl.oz.
$1^1/_4$	cups	310 ml
$1^1/_2$	cups	375 ml
$1^3/_4$	cups	440 ml
2	cups	500 ml
3	cups	750 ml
4	cups	1 litre
1 000ml		1 litre
$^1/_8$	tsp (teaspoon)	1 ml
$^1/_4$	tsp	2 ml
$^1/_2$	tsp	3 ml
1	tsp	5 ml
2	tsps	10 ml
3	tsps	15 ml
1	D (dessertspoon)	10 ml
1	T (tablespoon)	12,5 ml
2	T	25 ml
3	T	37,5 ml
4	T	50 ml
5	T	62,5 ml
6	T	75 ml

LIQUID CAPACITY

1	fluid ounce	30 ml
2	fluid ounces	60 ml
5	fluid ounces/1 gill	150 ml
$^1/_4$	pint	150 ml
8	fluid ounces/1 cup	250 ml
$^1/_2$	pint	300 ml
$^3/_4$	pint	450 ml
20	fluid ounces	600 ml
1	pint	600 ml
$1^1/_2$	pints	900 ml
2	pints/1 quart	1 200 ml
2	pints	1,2 litres
3	pints	1,8 litres
4	pints	2,5 litres
8	pints/1 gallon	5 litres

OVEN TEMPERATURES

Fahrenheit (°F)	Celcius (°C)	Gas Mark
Very Low		
200	100	$^1/_8$
225	110	$^1/_4$
250	120	$^1/_2$
Low		
275	140	1
300	150	2
325	160	3
Moderate		
350	180	4
375	190	5
400	200	6
High		
425	220	7
450	230	8
475	240	9
Very High		
500	260	10

CAKE PAN SIZES

5 inches		125 mm
6 inches		150 mm
7 inches		180 mm
8 inches		200 mm
9 inches		230 mm
10 inches		250 mm
11 inches		280 mm
12 inches		300 mm

SEE PRESERVES, PAGE 99

Note: When bottling diabetic jams and preserves, rather use several small jars, rather than one or two large ones. Once opened, storage time is limited, even in the refrigerator. There is a new product on the market, *Make-a-jam*, which will enable the diabetic to prepare small quantities of jam, with the simple addition of a quantity of powder.

Make-a-jam comes in 200 g packets and consists of fructose, food starch, thickeners, sodium cyclamate, acesulfame k, caramel for colour, and sorbic acid.

Make-a-jam lets you make jams, marmalades, chutneys and sauces in miinutes. Simply cook the fruit until soft, add water to make up to 250 ml, and bring to the boil. Stir in 50 g powder, and leave to set. Store in refrigerator.

INDEX

Apple and sprout salad 56
Apple triangles 72
Apricot and pineapple jam 96
Baked apricot pudding 69
Baked whole fish with mint
  vinaigrette 23
Baked eggs 9
Baked haddock with tomatoes and baby
  marrows 21
Banana and date pudding 73
Basic white sauce 92
Bean sprout stir-fry 42
Beef and bean casserole 28
Braised celery with peppers 43
Brinjal and rice bake 40
Brinjal pâté 16
Broccoli and cheese soup 17
Cabbage roll-ups 63
Carrot and tomato soup 13
Chicken and bread-cube salad 55
Chicken and mushroom pizza 61
Chicken and pea cobbler 36
Chicken and rice ring 39
Chicken asparagus rolls 33
Chicken breast fillets with rosemary 35
Chicken with artichokes and potatoes 35
Chicken, potato and spinach soup 14
Chocolate sauce 89
Christmas fruit-cake 104
Christmas mince pies 106
Christmas pudding 103
Cinnamon biscuits 84
Citrus Christmas mincemeat 107
Coq au vin 33
Cornish pasties 62
Country vegetable soup 13
Cream substitute 90
Crêpes au poisson 15
Crunchy hazel-nut mounds 86
Curried apple coleslaw 55
Curried mixed vegetables 45
Curry sauce 91
Diabetic cookie-press biscuits 80
Diabetic cup-cakes 75
Diabetic custard 89
Diabetic mayonnaise 93
Egg noodles with asparagus and poppy
  seeds 38
Fish and potato Frittata 9
French dressing 93
Frosted chocolate squares 76
Garlic and parsley dressing 90
Granadilla cream 71

Granary loaf 79
Grapefruit, apple and pear mix 11
Green tomato chutney 99
Green yoghurt dressing 90
Hake with pasta shells 40
Haricot beans with pumpkin sauce 50
Home-made beef stock 26
Home-made chicken stock 34
Home-made fish stock 20
Home-made tomato sauce 90
Home-made vegetable stock 44
Hot orange chutney 99
Indian pork chops 25
Kipper pâté 16
Lamb kebabs 25
Leek and ricotta money-bags 67
Lentil loaf 49
Lentil moussaka 53
Lettuce, olive and orange salad 57
Marinated T-bone steaks 25
Mealie-meal crumpets 11
Mexican chilli bean pizza 61
Mint sauce 90
Mixed bean Ratatouille 51
Muesli 10
Mushroom and lentil pâté 16
Mushroom meat patties 27
Mushroom soup 17
New potato salad 57
No-bake milk tart 69
Oat and raisin cookies 76
Oaty burgers 28
Onion relish 95
Open sandwiches 60
Orange and lemon marmalade 94
Peach cheesecake 70
Pear and orange jam 96
Pearled barley and lentil pilaff 51
Pickled garlic 98
Pickled mushrooms 99
Pizza tomato sauce 59
Poached hake with mushroom sauce 20
Pork stir-fry 31
Prune and duck casserole 36
Pumpkin soufflé 46
Queen of puddings 70
Raisin and oat bread 78
Red kidney bean slaw 56
Rhubarb and apple jam 96
Rice-stuffed kingklip 19
Roast duck with pear stuffing 37
Roast lamb with fresh herbs 31
Roast turkey 101

Salad and potato pie 59
Sausage and bean stew 50
Sesame pork schnitzels 27
Shredded wheat salad 54
Sole with crumb topping 19
Spanish omelette 66
Spicy broccoli with puréed pepper 43
Spicy salad dressing 91
Spicy bran muffins 80
Spinach and ricotta pizza 65
Spinach-stuffed mushrooms 14
Strawberry jam 95
Strawberry sauce 89
Strawberry-pineapple cheesecake 73
Striped green glory 68
Stuffed peppers 47
Sugar-free carrot cake 81
Sugarless banana bread 85
Sunflower rice salad 55
Sweet and sour meatballs 29
Sweet fruit tartlets 83
Tangy barbecue sauce 93
Thick celery soup 13
Thick lentil soup 50
Thirty-day health muffins 84
Three-fruit marmalade 96
Tuna and bean salad 49
Tuna fish cakes 22
Tuna-stuffed potatoes 21
Twisted pasta with lentils 41
Uncooked spicy cucumber pickles 99
Valentine biscuits 109
Vanilla ice-cream 72
Vanilla sandwich cake with creamy
  frosting 84
Vegetable pizza 61
Vegetable hot-pot 46
Vegetarian jambalaya 41
Whipped topping 90
Wholewheat banana cookies 85
Wholewheat bean and cheese loaf 79
Wholewheat chocolate apple cake 75
Wholewheat choux puffs 82
Wholewheat flaky pastry 102
Wholewheat french toast 10
Wholewheat pizza crust 66
Wholewheat plait 78
Wholewheat potato rolls 79
Wholewheat shortbread 108
Wholewheat yoghurt scones 76
Wrapped pork with prunes 30

© Vlaeberg Publishers, P.O. Box 15034, Vlaeberg 8018, South Africa

First edition. First impression 1993

Production and design: Wim Reinders & Associates
Cover design: Abdul Amien
Typeset and reproduction: Hirt & Carter, Cape Town

ISBN 0-947461-29-9